ATLAS OF
Cancer Mortality
IN ENGLAND AND WALES

1968–1978

ATLAS OF
Cancer Mortality
IN ENGLAND AND WALES
1968–1978

M. J. Gardner
P. D. Winter
C. P. Taylor
E. D. Acheson

Medical Research Council
Environmental Epidemiology Unit
(University of Southampton)
Southampton General Hospital
Southampton, UK

A Wiley Medical Publication

JOHN WILEY & SONS
Chichester · New York · Brisbane · Toronto · Singapore

Library of Congress Cataloging in Publication Data:

Main entry under title:

Atlas of cancer mortality in England and Wales, 1968–
    1978.

   (A Wiley medical publication)
   1. Cancer—England—Mortality—Atlases. 2. Cancer
—Wales—Mortality—Atlases. I. Gardner, M. J.
II. Series. [DNLM: 1. Neoplasms—Mortality—England.
2. Neoplasms—Mortality—Wales. QZ 16 A881]
RC279.G7A78   1983   614.5'999   83-5961
ISBN 0 471 90042 7

British Library Cataloguing in Publication Data:

Atlas of cancer mortality in England and Wales,
    1968–1978.
    1. Cancer—England—Mortality—Maps
    I. Gardner, M.J.
    912'130464   RC279.G7

    ISBN 0 471 90042 7

Typeset by Pintail Studios Ltd., Ringwood, Hampshire.
Reproduction origination by Sayl Reproductions, Southampton.
Printed in Great Britain by BAS Printers Limited,
Over Wallop, Stockbridge, Hampshire.

Contents

Preface

In the years that preceded the First World War, knowledge of the causes of cancer grew almost entirely as a result of recognizing that different types of cancer occurred characteristically in men and women who were engaged in a particular occupation or lived in a particular part of the world. Important knowledge was obtained in this way which has stood the test of time, some even becoming the foundation stone on which our knowledge of chemical carcinogenesis was built. Progress, however, was slow. Quantitative data were usually lacking and advance depended, for the most part, on the acumen of individuals who were struck by seeing a cluster of patients with a particular type of cancer and a common background of occupation, place of residence, or cultural behaviour.

Later, when Stocks and his successors began to apply the rigorous techniques that had been evolved for the study of infectious disease to the study of cancer, little attention was paid to their results. For by then, Yamagiwa and Ishikawa had produced cancer experimentally by painting tar on a rabbit's ear and the potential of laboratory experiment had captured the imagination of the scientific world. Observational data, that had not been obtained by experiment, were liable to misinterpretation, because of the difficulty of distinguishing between an association reflecting cause and effect and a trivial one due to an incidental association between the observed characteristic and the true cause; and there seemed little point in worrying about them, as it was confidently believed that the mechanism by which all cancer was caused would soon be discovered.

The results of laboratory experiment have indeed been impressive and there are once again grounds for thinking that the hope that has been for so long unfulfilled may indeed be realized within the next decade. Meanwhile, however, interest in epidemiological observations has revived and it is now widely appreciated that they have a useful part to play, not only in identifying causes with sufficient certainty to justify preventive action and suggesting hypotheses for laboratory investigation, but also in testing the relevance of laboratory results for the human situation. This revival has brought with it a new interest in the mapping of cancer incidence and mortality both broadly throughout the world and, in detail, within each country.

On a world wide scale the differences in incidence that have been observed encourage the belief that all the common types of cancer are largely avoidable, in the sense that it should be possible to reduce the risk of developing each type by at least a half and often by 80 per cent or more. Within one country, like Britain, social and environmental features are unlikely to differ enough between different parts to lead to such gross differences in incidence, but the observations that can be made have two notable advantages. First, the information available about the characteristics of the population and the diseases they experience is more extensive and more precise than that available generally between countries. Secondly, the common cultural background that is more or less uniform throughout the country makes it easier to detect distortions due, for example, to concentrations of hazardous industry in specific areas.

Professor Acheson and Dr. Gardner have built up a centre in Southampton which has become internationally known for its precision and economy in the handling of epidemiological data. The cancer atlas that they and their colleagues have produced has had to use mortality rather than incidence data, since the latter are still not collected in a sufficiently uniform way to make geographical comparisons within Britain reliable; but area differences in fatality rates are unlikely to be great enough to have affected materially the results. The atlas is a monument not only to their own work but also to that of the Central Office of Population Censuses and Surveys and Registrars throughout the country, without whose attention to detail the records would not be worth compiling. It is a fortunate accident that the atlas should be published in the centenary year of the death of William Farr, whose work as Superintendent of the Statistical Department of the General Register Office set the standards which have made such compilations of practical research value and has inspired medical statisticians to use them ever since.

Sir Richard Doll

Contents

Maps

Tables and Graphs

Contents

Introduction

Mapping of disease rates is a helpful way of displaying the available data to enable spatial patterns, such as clusters of neighbouring areas with similar rates or gradients of rates across the country to be visually apparent. By so doing, the contrast of areas with low and high rates, in respect of their environmental and other characteristics, may lead to the development of hypotheses about causal factors which are responsible for any differences.

The geographical distribution of disease has been displayed by the use of maps for over a century on local, national and international scales. For England and Wales three reports by Stocks in the late 1930s included maps at county level of death rates from 17 types of cancer during the period 1921–30 (1). Later, an atlas of mortality for the United Kingdom was produced by Howe covering the years 1954–58 and 1959–63 (2). It included maps for 4 sites of cancer — namely, lung, stomach, breast and uterus — which showed striking, and different, geographical distributions. The areas used were the individual Metropolitan Boroughs and County Boroughs and the aggregated Urban Districts and aggregated Rural Districts within each of the Administrative Counties. More recently, for deaths occurring during the years 1969–73, maps have been produced for 16 cancers on a regional scale — using the 10 standard regions of England and Wales (3).

To enable a more detailed local investigation for a larger number of sites of cancer, we have used information obtained from the Office of Population Censuses and Surveys on computer tape for the years 1968–78. From these data, death rates for an extensive list of different cancers have been calculated for each of the 1366 Local Authority areas as constituted in 1971, as well as aggregated areas such as Counties. Maps of the geographical distribution of these cancers are shown in this volume, and the mortality rates upon which they are based are available separately (4). A second volume presenting maps of individual causes of death other than from cancer in a similar manner is being prepared. The mode of presentation has been influenced by that of the United States atlas for 3056 counties (5).

We are using the mortality data in other ways. Thus, as well as any subjective visual impressions which may be gained from studying the maps, correlational studies with measured social and environmental factors are being undertaken to search for clues to causation. For example, in preliminary investigations with particular reference to occupation, we have found that death rates from nasal cancer are related to the proportion of the population working in the furniture and leather industries (6), and that mortality from pleural mesothelioma was high in areas of known extensive usage of asbestos in the relevant past (7). These associations were known previously, but indicate that this approach to the possible identification of causes may prove fruitful. Thus Stocks, in his studies some 40 years ago (8), demonstrated the strong relationship between high cancer of the stomach death rates and indices of poor social conditions, which still persists.

Should the reasons why persons living in some areas have a lower risk of cancer than those in other areas be elucidated, then the implications for prevention and health education would become clear.

Methods

We obtained extracts of all primary death records for the period 1959–79 on computer tape from the Office of Population Censuses and Surveys for England and Wales. These extracts included five items of information on each death — year of death, sex, age at death, the Local Authority area code for place of residence at the time of death, and the code number of the certified underlying cause of death according to the International Classification of Diseases (ICD). None of the deceased persons can be identified individually.

There are problems associated with amalgamating the mortality data over the whole of the 21-year period by cause and area for at least three important reasons. First, there have been modifications to the ICD which has passed through its seventh, eighth and ninth Revisions during this time, and these have not always allowed continuity of classification by cause of death. Secondly, there was a major reorganisation of Local Authority area boundaries during 1974, and other changes have occurred continually throughout the period on a smaller scale. For each death registered from 1974 onwards, however, we obtained also the area of residence coded to the pre-1974 boundaries. Thirdly, population figures for each Local Authority area by age and sex are only available for the Census years 1961 and 1971, but during the period there will have been changes in population structure due to births, deaths and migration. Because of these difficulties we decided to include only deaths which occurred during the years 1968–78 in the death rates calculated for the purpose of this atlas. These eleven years span the complete duration of the eighth Revision of the ICD (9). The boundaries used are those of the Local Authority areas and Counties as at the 1971 Census. The population figures used for each of the areas by sex and age are also as at the 1971 Census, and are those used in the area analysis for 1969–73 (3).

The mortality rates by sex and type of cancer for each Local Authority area and County were calculated relative to England and Wales as a whole. The index used is the Standardised Mortality Ratio (SMR), which incorporates an adjustment for differences between the age structure of the local and national populations (3). The SMR is scaled so that the ratio for England and Wales is 100. An age-standardised death rate for each area can be obtained by multiplying the local SMR by the overall death rate from that cancer in England and Wales. Areas with SMRs numerically less than 100 thus have age-standardised death rates lower than the national overall figure, and vice-versa. Confidence intervals for the SMRs were calculated assuming that the number of observed deaths in an area followed a Poisson distribution. A local SMR was determined to be significantly different from England and Wales at the 5% level of statistical significance if the 95% confidence interval for that local SMR did not contain 100.

During the years 1968–78 there were 1,320,614 deaths certified with cancer (ICD Numbers 140–209) as the underlying cause registered to persons in England and Wales. This is an annual figure of some 120,000, which represents about 20 per cent of the total deaths each year. Maps of these deaths by cause are presented in two sections. The first contains maps for all causes combined, all cancers combined and sites of cancer for which, in general, the largest numbers of deaths occurred (over 10,000 in each sex during the 11 years). For each of these sites, for each sex where appropriate, a map is presented illustrating separately the low and high mortality places among the 1366 Local Authority areas. An exception is made by the inclusion of mesothelioma of the pleura with high areas only being shown. This section includes 25 maps – 11 for men and 14 for women. The second section includes 44 maps (22 for men and 22 for women) for a selection of the remaining cancers, some of which are combinations of separate ICD categories. These show the distribution of death rates on a County scale rather than for smaller geographical areas, due to the smaller numbers of deaths involved. For this reason also the county of Rutland has been merged with Leicestershire (as it was in the post-1974 re-organisation), and Wales has been amalgamated into its two Standard Regions. Wales I contains the counties of Brecon, Carmarthen, Glamorgan and Monmouth, with the remaining Welsh counties constituting Wales II. As a consequence 47 areas are mapped in Section 2.

In Section 1, six types of area are colour-shaded on each map according to combinations of 4 conditions – namely, (a) whether the local SMR is less than or greater than 100 (i.e., whether the local age-standardised death rate is less than or greater than the national overall rate), (b) whether the SMR if it is less (greater) than 100 is in the bottom (top) tenth or not of the distribution among the 1366 Local Authority areas, (c) whether or not the SMR, in the statistical sense, is significantly less (greater) than 100, and (d) areas where fewer than 4 deaths from a particular cause occurred during the 11 years but the SMR was over 100 are not shaded on the corresponding map, even if the SMR was in the top tenth. The third criteria, (c), has been incorporated to lessen the emphasis placed on low or high rates in areas with limited size of population. This is done to reduce the attention attracted to areas where the numerical basis of the calculated SMR is less reliable than in areas with larger populations. Three different densities of green are used to represent areas with low SMRs, and three varying reds for areas with high SMRs – with resemblance to the "traffic-light" system. All the remaining areas, with SMRs which do not satisfy one of the criteria shown on the legends of the maps, are left unshaded. The County boundaries have been over-printed to assist in the identification of specific areas.

In Section 2, four types of area are colour-shaded on each map. The particular colour, in this instance, directly indicates the range of numerical values within which the area's SMR lies. The divisions used, symmetrical around an SMR of 100, are: under 75, 75–89, 90–109, 110–124, 125 and over. As a contrast to the colours used in Section 1, two different densities of blue and orange are used for the maps in Section 2 to represent the lower and higher ranges respectively. Areas with SMRs within 10 per cent either above or below the national average are left white. Since areas with larger population have been used in this section of the atlas the criterion of statistical significance has been omitted, even though the overall numbers of deaths from each cancer in the country are smaller. However, attention has been paid to it in the later description of the maps, and detailed information is available with the complete data (4).

The maps have been produced by computer using the ICL 2970 at the University of Southampton. A version of the GIMMS program (10) was used to generate black and white shaded output on a Calcomp plotter. This was then photographed, reduced and colour printed. The boundaries were reproduced from the digitised boundaries of the Local Authority areas and Counties obtained on magnetic tape from the Department of the Environment.

Following the map sections of the atlas there is a one-page summary of some features of the deaths from each cancer. These include the numbers of deaths and the death rates per million population by age groups for each sex in tabular and in graphical form for England and Wales as a whole. The age groups shown are the same as those used to calculate the local area SMRs. For each cause of death in Section 1 the distribution of the SMRs among the 1366 Local Authority areas in tenths, the number of areas with no deaths from the particular cancer during the 11 years, and the number of areas in each of the mapping categories are also given. For each cancer in section 2 the number of areas in each mapping category is tabulated, together with the lowest and highest SMRs and the number of areas where no deaths occurred.

On the "contents" pages of this atlas the full description of each type of cancer and its 3 or 4 digit code number according to the International Classification of Diseases (9) are given. In subsequent pages a shortened title is sometimes utilised, but in all cases the complete expanded meaning is implied. Throughout, the more widely understood word "cancer" has been substituted for the technical term "malignant neoplasm".

Maps giving the names of the 1366 Local Authority areas and the new post-1974 Districts are shown at the end of the Atlas, and have been reproduced from originals produced by the Department of the Environment.

Interpretation

Before drawing any firm conclusions about whether an area has low or high mortality from a particular type or types of cancer, the reader's attention is drawn to the following considerations:

1. The cause of death on which the death rates are based is the underlying cause of death as coded from the diagnosis written on the death certificate. This diagnosis is not always easy to make and is known to be subject to errors, particularly in the elderly (11, 12). Also, there may be variations in death certification practice between areas.

2. The assignment of area of residence for any individual death is generally straightforward, except for persons who die in institutions. In some of these latter instances, where institutions are termed as long-stay, there are coding rules which allocate deaths to the area of the institution rather than to the area of usual residence of the individual.

One area uniquely affected in this way is Stone Rural District in Staffordshire which appears as high for cancer mortality on 19 of the 23 maps in Section 1. This is due to the presence of a terminal care hospital for cancer patients of all ages in a district of relatively small population. Many persons who died in this institution, and whose deaths were coded to the area, had their home residence in other neighbouring Local Authority areas. No other area appears as high on more than 11 maps.

3. The population figures used to calculate the mortality indices are based on the 1971 Census. Migration during the period 1968 to 1978 could therefore influence the accuracy of the calculated death rates.

4. Migration over a longer period of time between birth and death may also influence the death rates for an area. Thus, for example, any patterns which are associated with causal factors operative in early life may be blurred or exaggerated by migration later in life. In addition, selective migration on ill health grounds, either long distance to retirement areas or from rural areas into towns to, for example, sheltered accommodation, may increase death rates in certain areas. A more detailed account of some effects of migration on area mortality is provided by Fox and Goldblatt (13).

If it is reasonable to assume that these and other such, possibly less obvious, influences are not greatly affecting the death rates for particular cancers and areas of interest, then it becomes pertinent to examine other reasons for the deficit or excess mortality. One such reason could be the result of any differential effects of treatment existing between areas. Although survival rates after diagnosis of cancer do vary between regions, the differences are relatively slight (14). Moreover, survival is not necessarily longest where mortality is lowest. Another related feature to bear in mind is that the maps represent deaths, and thus all cases of cancer which occur are not included. For some sites, such as oesophagus, stomach and lung, prognosis is relatively unfavourable and mortality more closely reflects incidence. For other sites, particularly cancers of the skin, but also cancers of the uterus and testis, survival after initial diagnosis is much better and this could affect the geographical patterns.

Other suggested explanatory factors which may be considered, in no special order, include:

(a) general external factors such as climate, soil and the quality of air and water,

(b) personal factors of individual behaviour, such as diet, smoking and reproductive/sexual behaviour,

(c) occupational and industrial environment of the individual and of the area, and

(d) genetic factors.

For a general discussion of the possible roles played by various factors in the causation of cancer the reader is referred to the book by Doll and Peto (15). In the following section, comments are limited to a description of the main features of the maps without any suggestive explanatory remarks.

Description of Maps

Some of the maps show clear and distinctive distributions of mortality, although there are others where little obvious geographical pattern emerges. In general terms it can be said that death rates from cancers of the breast, ovary, brain, melanoma of the skin and non-Hodgkin's lymphoma were lower in the north; while mortality from cancers of the buccal cavity, pharynx, stomach, rectum, cervix and kidney tended to be lower in the south. There were high rates from cancer of the oesophagus in Lancashire and among women in Wales, and from cancer of the lung in some of the conurbations.

For the maps in Section 1 the following more detailed features are noticeable:

All causes of death   The general areas of low mortality are in the south and east, although there are a number of London boroughs with high rates for men. The largest clusters of areas with high mortality for both sexes are south Lancashire, the West Riding of Yorkshire, Tyneside, Durham and south Wales. There are a number of instances of adjacent areas having contrasting rates in both sexes — for example, in Dorset. These tend to be high in towns and low in neighbouring rural districts — this is a situation where interpretation may be complicated by problems with residential coding and the effects of differential migration of the sick. (See paragraphs 2 and 4 in the section on "Interpretation".)

All cancers   Areas of low mortality are scattered throughout the country for both men and women, with a noticeable concentration in the southern part of the West Riding of Yorkshire contrary to its high total mortality. The regions with high rates are London, south Lancashire and Tyneside, plus a number of areas in the Midlands for men only.

Oesophagus   An area in the central part of the country (south West Riding of Yorkshire, Derbyshire, Nottinghamshire and Leicestershire) has mainly low rates in both sexes, as does London. There is a suggestion of high rates in parts of Cornwall and Devon, and for men only in the south of Kent and in Rutland. For women there is a cluster of areas with high rates on the Cheshire/Staffordshire border, together with high levels in Wales — particularly in the northern coastal strip.

Stomach   Among predominantly low rates in a region covering East Anglia, central south England and the south-west, the east of London is noticeably different with a cluster of boroughs having high rates. The well-known high rate in Wales is shown to be a fairly widespread feature, affecting a large proportion of the constituent Local Authority areas. The same is true for Staffordshire, south Lancashire, parts of Cumberland and the West Riding of Yorkshire, Durham and Tyneside in both sexes.

Large intestine   London, for both sexes, has many boroughs which experienced low rates. The other prominent feature is the west of Lancashire, with a number of areas having high female mortality in contrast to men for whom areas with both low and high rates are found. For men and women there are some high rates around Tyneside.

Rectum   Rates in London and the south-east are mainly low, particularly for men. In the Midlands, south Lancashire and the West

Riding of Yorkshire there are a number of areas with high rates, and this is so for men around Tyneside.

Pancreas   The difficulties associated with the diagnosis of cancer of the pancreas are probably greater than for most other sites, and this may be a reason for the apparent lack of any clear pattern. Virtually all over the country areas with low and high rates are intermixed.

Lung   In both sexes the predominant feature is of low mortality in the less densely populated areas away from the major cities. Interesting differences between the sexes are the more widespread occurrence of high rates around south Lancashire for men than for women, and the contrast of high mortality for men with low mortality for women around the Staffordshire / Warwickshire / Worcestershire border. A further difference between the sexes is the spread of mainly high rates in areas surrounding London for women, but of low rates for men. Throughout Wales, including the more urban south, rates are generally low.

Breast (women)   The main areas of low mortality are in the north of the country including Lancashire, Yorkshire and Durham. On the contrary the south-east and Midlands, with occasional exceptions, have areas with high rates.

Cervix   Low rates predominate throughout London and the south-east of the country. In contrast, women in north and south-west Wales, Lancashire, the West Riding of Yorkshire and Tyneside have increased mortality from this site of cancer in many areas. There are also high rates in parts of Cornwall and Nottinghamshire.

Other Uterus   Mortality from this site shows a mixed distribution by area with no obvious outstanding features. Some areas in the south-west of England, in south-west Wales and central England have high rates.

Ovary   There are areas of low mortality in Lancashire and south Wales in particular, and to a lesser extent in the north-east. Areas with high rates are found mainly in the south coastal counties, but also occur in Cheshire and the West and East Ridings of Yorkshire.

Bladder   Low rates are found in south Wales and the south-west, and for men in other scattered areas of the country. For both men and women there are areas of high mortality in London and its surrounds, as well as in parts of Lancashire and the West Riding of Yorkshire. However, the precise areas which have high rates rarely correspond in the two sexes.

Prostate   For this site areas with low rates predominate in the north, north-east and south Wales, but are not exclusively found in these regions. Many of the areas with high rates are located in the south-west and south-east.

Mesothelioma of the pleura   There are areas of high mortality for men around some of the major ports and naval dockyards. For women there are clusters of high areas in Lancashire, the West Riding of Yorkshire and near Nottingham. For both sexes there are a number of boroughs in east London with high rates. Among the 1,366 Local Authority areas, 916 for men and 1,133 for women had no deaths from this cause during 1968–78, and so a large proportion of the areas not colour-shaded for each sex had zero rates.

For the cancers included in Section 2 of the atlas, on a County rather than Local Authority area basis, the following brief observations can be made from the maps:

Buccal Cavity   For each sex, this cancer has a marked south to north distribution. Rates, with only few exceptions, are low in the south and high in the north. For women, there are a number of adjoining counties with noticeably high rates on the central eastern coast.

Pharynx   The areas with low rates, for both men and women, are predominantly in the south and east of the country. Counties with high rates are found in the north-east with a band in the central west. There are particularly high rates for women in Wales, which is similar to cancers of the oesophagus and stomach.

Liver   There are a number of counties stretching across the south of England with low rates for men, but for both sexes there are low areas scattered further north. The high rates for men in Northumberland, Lancashire and Warwickshire derive from the large cities, with Greater London having high rates for men predominantly in its central boroughs.

Gall bladder   The suggestion for each sex is that areas of low mortality are away from the central part of the country, but this is less striking for women. There are four central counties – Warwickshire, Oxfordshire, Northamptonshire and Nottinghamshire – as well as Durham which have high rates for both men and women.

Nose   Counties with low and high rates are scattered around the country, but Buckinghamshire, Dorset and West Suffolk have rates in the highest group for both men and women. The high mortality for men in Buckinghamshire has been alluded to earlier, and is associated with the furniture industry around High Wycombe.

Larynx   For men the counties with low rates are predominantly in the south and east, with high rates further north. Areas with low and high rates show no particular geographical pattern for women, with only Lancashire and Surrey having statistically significant high rates.

Bone   Counties with low mortality are spread around the country with little distinctive grouping. For women there are high rates in some eastern counties, with Huntingdonshire and Bedfordshire also having raised rates for men. Additionally, Northumberland and Lancashire, particularly in the large towns, have high rates for both sexes.

Connective and other soft tissue   For both men and women the areas with low rates are dispersed, but the counties with highest rates seem to be predominantly in the south. There is little important statistical variation, however, only Hampshire for women having significantly raised mortality.

Melanoma of the skin   In both sexes there is a distinct pattern of counties in the north of the country having low rates and those in the south having high rates. With the sole exception of the Isle of Wight for women, south coast counties all have above national average mortality for men and women.

Other skin   These cancers have a different geographical distribution to melanoma of the skin, with low areas being mainly in the south and south-east. Counties with high rates are in the west, including Wales, the north and the north-east particularly for women.

Vulva and other female genital organs   There is a tendency for counties in the south-east to have low rates, as well as three of the most northern counties. An area from south-west to north-east across the country has a number of counties with high rates.

Testis   Although areas with low and high rates are somewhat interspersed, the counties with the highest rates are in the south-east and East Anglia. The rates in Durham and Lancashire are particularly low.

Kidney and other urinary organs   Except in the north, low rates are found in areas covering most of the country for both sexes. Durham and Northumberland (in the latter case, particularly Tyneside) have high rates for both men and women, but a number of neighbouring counties also have raised mortality among women.

Brain   Although not exclusively so, more areas with low rates are found on moving northwards. All parts of Lincolnshire, together with Leicestershire and Rutland, have decreased mortality for both men and women. The most prominent feature of these maps, and particularly for men, is the concentration of areas with high rates in the south.

Thyroid gland   The areas of low and high rates are generally interspersed, and there is little similarity about the distributions for men and women. Moreover, there is very little statistically significant variation between the counties.

Unspecified site   The main areas with low rates are coincident for men and women, although they are geographically scattered. There is a collection of counties between Warwickshire and Greater London with high rates, and a more detailed look at the available information reveals raised mortality in Birmingham and in many of the constituent boroughs of London. Deaths assigned to this classification are mainly from cancers of multiple sites where the primary site is not specified, and it is unlikely in this case that the geographical pattern has any biological meaning.

Non-Hodgkin's lymphoma   There is a clear tendency for low rates among counties in the north, with high mortality being found predominantly in the south. The difference is marked and occurs for both men and women, with only occasional exceptions.

Hodgkin's disease   The geographical distribution is mixed, but there are a number of counties with contiguous boundaries which have similar rates. In central southern counties the rates are predominantly low, with bands of higher mortality running across the middle of the country for each sex. Rates are particularly high in north Wales.

Multiple myeloma   There are low rates in a number of counties for each sex in the central area of the country, with high rates being prominent in the south. Lancashire has low mortality for both men and women.

Leukaemias   These cancers have mixed geographical distributions with little obvious pattern. For acute lymphatic leukaemia there are high rates for both men and women in Derbyshire and East Sussex, with Lincolnshire (Holland) having the highest rate in each sex for chronic lymphatic leukaemia. Rates for acute myeloid leukaemia are lower in the north than in the south for men, but a more heterogeneous pattern exists for women. Chronic myeloid leukaemia has counties with low and high rates in various parts of the country, although Dorset and the North Riding of Yorkshire have raised mortality for both sexes.

Acknowledgements

We would like to thank the Office of Population Censuses and Surveys for making available the basic material on the deaths which occurred during the years involved, and the Head Office of the Medical Research Council for their help during the negotiation period. Without their co-operation the production of this Atlas would not have been possible.

The Computing Service of the University of Southampton have contributed generously in advice during the computing work involved in processing the data and drawing the maps, and we are grateful to them.

The Map Library of the Department of the Environment kindly agreed to the reproduction of two of their detailed maps which markedly aid the identification of areas with low and high cancer mortality. The two maps are Crown copyright and are reproduced with the permission of the Controller of Her Majesty's Stationery Office.

We would like to thank also our colleagues in the MRC Environmental Epidemiology Unit who have contributed in various ways.

References

1. Stocks P. (1936, 1937 and 1939). Distribution in England and Wales of cancer of various sites. *Annual Reports of the British Empire Cancer Campaign*, **13**, 239–280; **14**, 198–223 and **16**, 308–343.

2. Howe G. M. (1970). *National Atlas of Disease Mortality in the United Kingdom*. London, Nelson.

3. Office of Population Censuses and Surveys (1981). *Area Mortality Decennial Supplement 1969–73, England and Wales*. Series DS, no. 4. London, HMSO.

4. Medical Research Council Environmental Epidemiology Unit. Lists of mortality by area, site and sex: 1968–78.

5. Mason T. J., McKay F. W., Hoover R., Blot W. J. and Fraumeni J. F. (1975). *Atlas of cancer mortality for U.S. Counties: 1950–1969*. Washington, U.S. Government Printing Office.

6. Gardner M. J., Winter P. D. and Acheson E. D. (1981). Variations in cancer mortality among local authority areas in England and Wales: relations with environmental factors and search for causes. *British Medical Journal*, **284**, 784–787.

7. Gardner M. J., Acheson E. D. and Winter P. D. (1982). Mesothelioma of the pleura in England and Wales during 1968–78. *British Journal of Cancer*, **46**, 81–88.

8. Stocks P. (1947). Regional and local differences in cancer death rates. *General Register Office, Studies on Medical and Population Subjects, No. 1*. London, HMSO.

9. World Health Organisation (1967). *International Classification of Diseases, Eighth Revision*. Geneva, WHO.

10. Waugh T. C. (1979). *GIMMS Reference Manual*. Program Library Unit, University of Edinburgh.

11. Cochrane A. L. and Moore F. (1981). Death certification from the epidemiological point of view. *Lancet, ii*, 742–743.

12. Cameron H. M. and McGoogan E. (1981). A prospective study of 1152 hospital autopsies: I. Inaccuracies in death certification. *Journal of Pathology*, **133**, 273–283.

13. Fox A. J. and Goldblatt, P. O. (1982). *Socio-demographic Mortality Differentials*. Office of Population Censuses and Surveys Series LS, no. 1. London, HMSO.

14. Office of Population Censuses and Surveys (1980). *Cancer Statistics: Survival*. Series MB1, no. 3. London, HMSO.

15. Doll R. and Peto R. (1981). *The Causes of Cancer*. Oxford, University Press.

Section 1

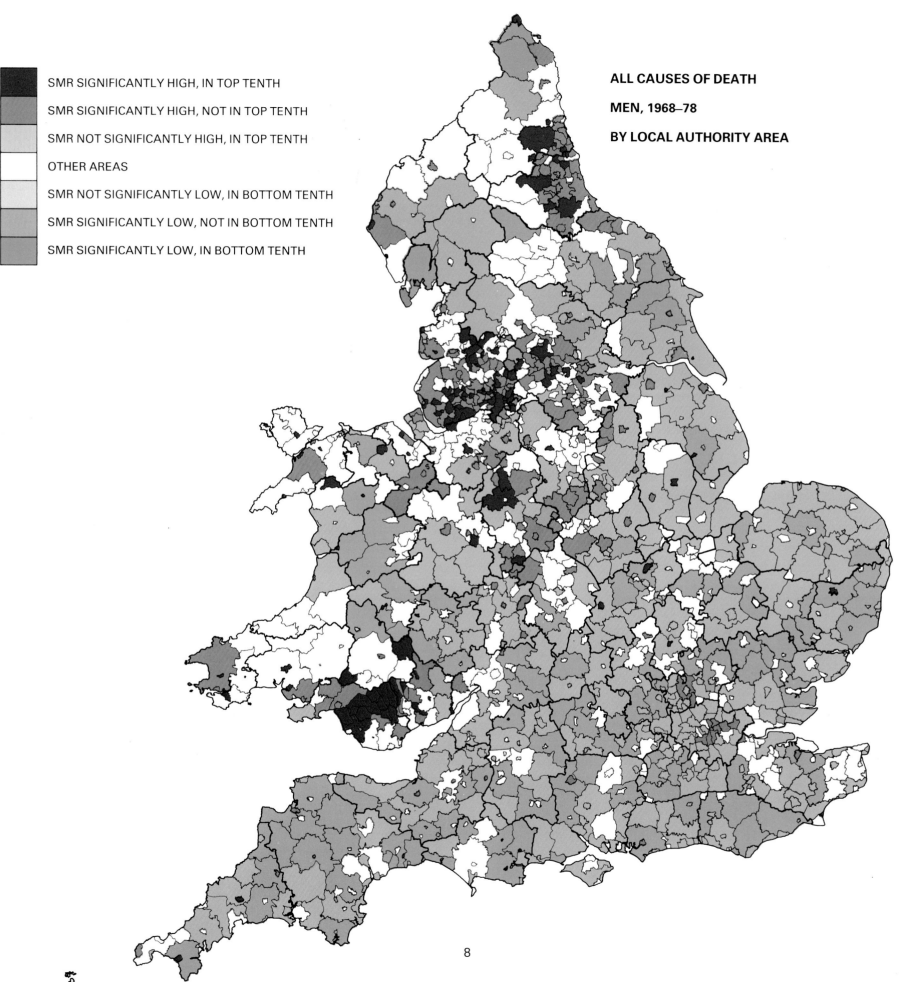

SMR SIGNIFICANTLY HIGH, IN TOP TENTH

SMR SIGNIFICANTLY HIGH, NOT IN TOP TENTH

SMR NOT SIGNIFICANTLY HIGH, IN TOP TENTH

OTHER AREAS

SMR NOT SIGNIFICANTLY LOW, IN BOTTOM TENTH

SMR SIGNIFICANTLY LOW, NOT IN BOTTOM TENTH

SMR SIGNIFICANTLY LOW, IN BOTTOM TENTH

ALL CAUSES OF DEATH

MEN, 1968–78

BY LOCAL AUTHORITY AREA

8

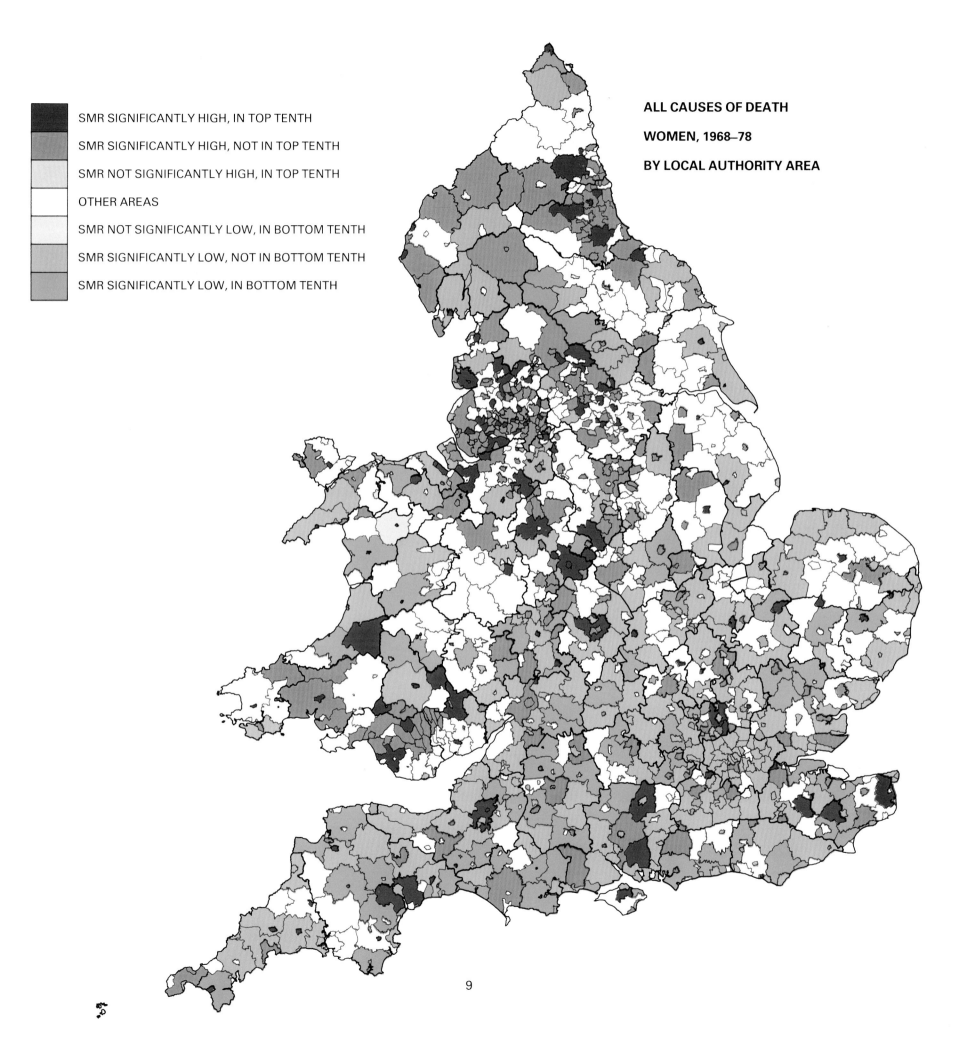

SMR SIGNIFICANTLY HIGH, IN TOP TENTH

SMR SIGNIFICANTLY HIGH, NOT IN TOP TENTH

SMR NOT SIGNIFICANTLY HIGH, IN TOP TENTH

OTHER AREAS

SMR NOT SIGNIFICANTLY LOW, IN BOTTOM TENTH

SMR SIGNIFICANTLY LOW, NOT IN BOTTOM TENTH

SMR SIGNIFICANTLY LOW, IN BOTTOM TENTH

ALL CAUSES OF DEATH

WOMEN, 1968–78

BY LOCAL AUTHORITY AREA

9

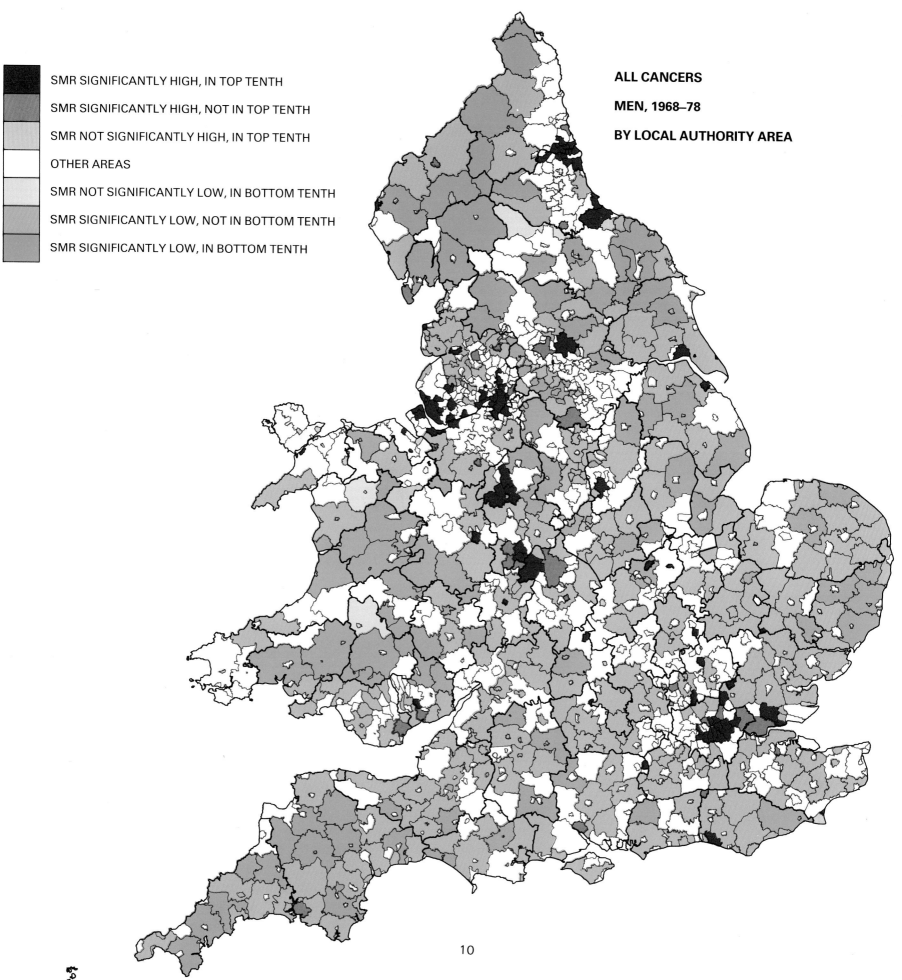

SMR SIGNIFICANTLY HIGH, IN TOP TENTH

SMR SIGNIFICANTLY HIGH, NOT IN TOP TENTH

SMR NOT SIGNIFICANTLY HIGH, IN TOP TENTH

OTHER AREAS

SMR NOT SIGNIFICANTLY LOW, IN BOTTOM TENTH

SMR SIGNIFICANTLY LOW, NOT IN BOTTOM TENTH

SMR SIGNIFICANTLY LOW, IN BOTTOM TENTH

ALL CANCERS

MEN, 1968–78

BY LOCAL AUTHORITY AREA

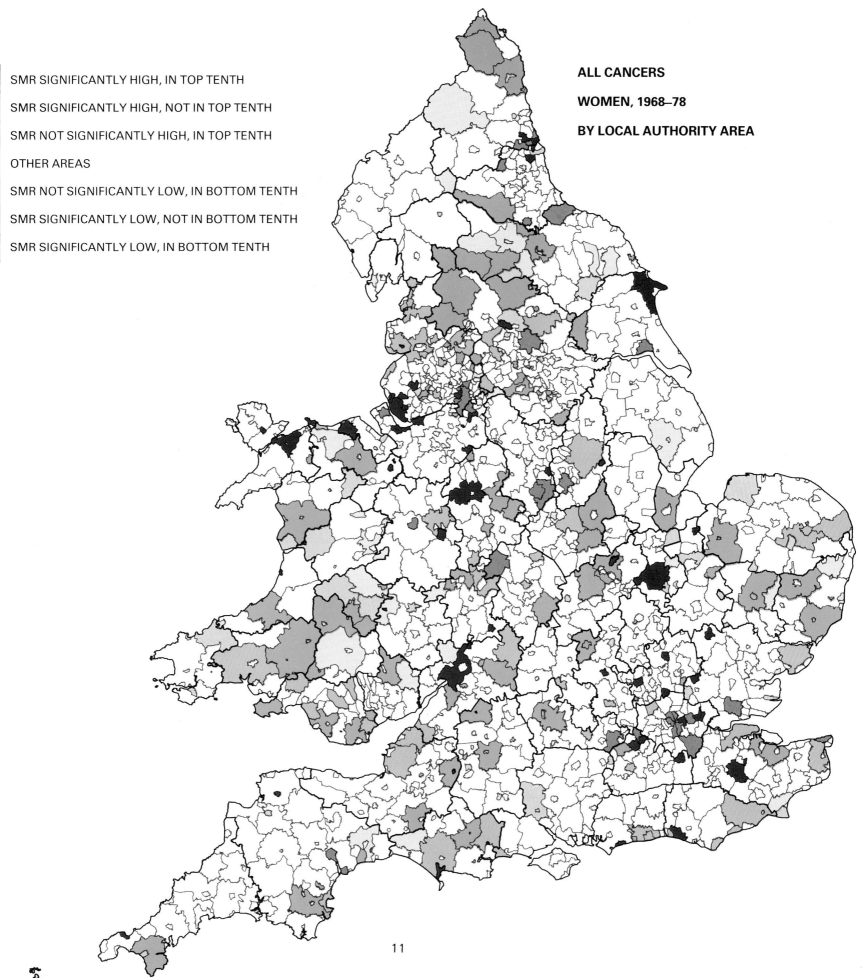

SMR SIGNIFICANTLY HIGH, IN TOP TENTH

SMR SIGNIFICANTLY HIGH, NOT IN TOP TENTH

SMR NOT SIGNIFICANTLY HIGH, IN TOP TENTH

OTHER AREAS

SMR NOT SIGNIFICANTLY LOW, IN BOTTOM TENTH

SMR SIGNIFICANTLY LOW, NOT IN BOTTOM TENTH

SMR SIGNIFICANTLY LOW, IN BOTTOM TENTH

ALL CANCERS

WOMEN, 1968–78

BY LOCAL AUTHORITY AREA

11

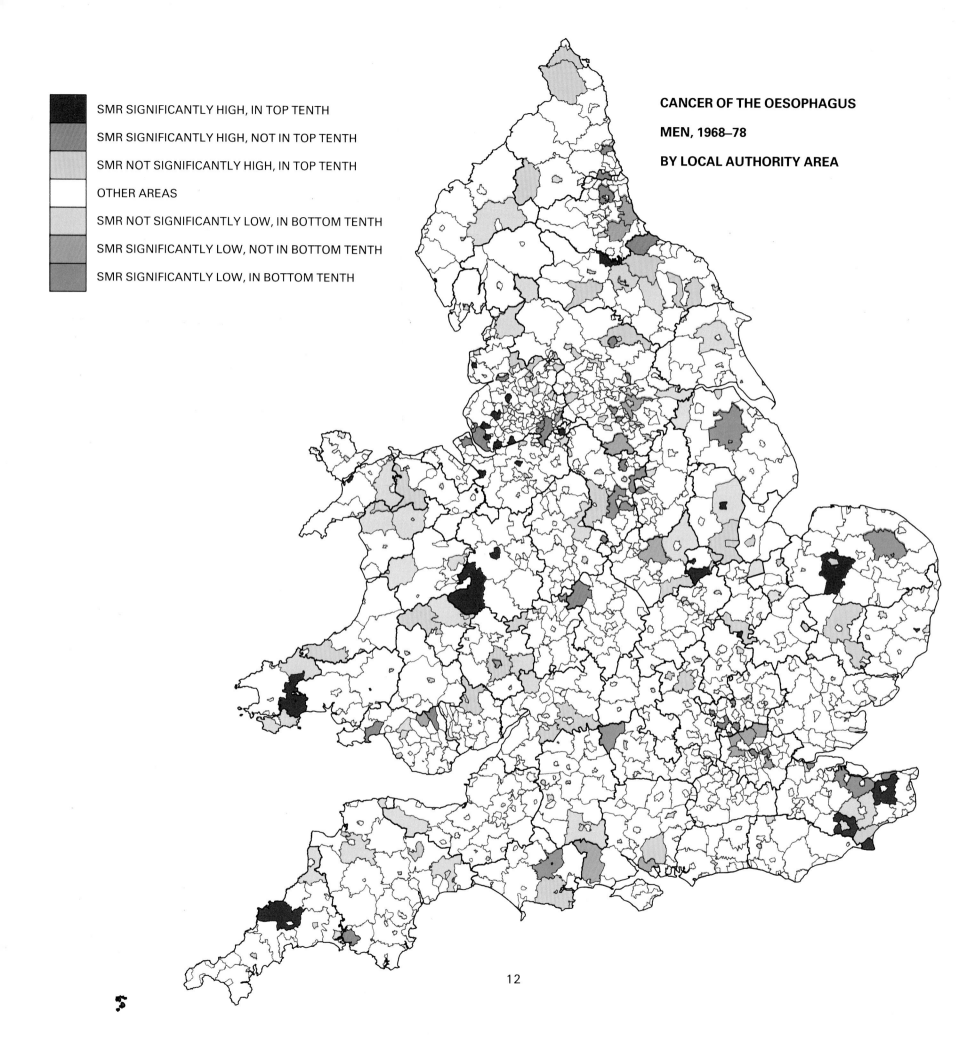

CANCER OF THE OESOPHAGUS

MEN, 1968–78

BY LOCAL AUTHORITY AREA

SMR SIGNIFICANTLY HIGH, IN TOP TENTH

SMR SIGNIFICANTLY HIGH, NOT IN TOP TENTH

SMR NOT SIGNIFICANTLY HIGH, IN TOP TENTH

OTHER AREAS

SMR NOT SIGNIFICANTLY LOW, IN BOTTOM TENTH

SMR SIGNIFICANTLY LOW, NOT IN BOTTOM TENTH

SMR SIGNIFICANTLY LOW, IN BOTTOM TENTH

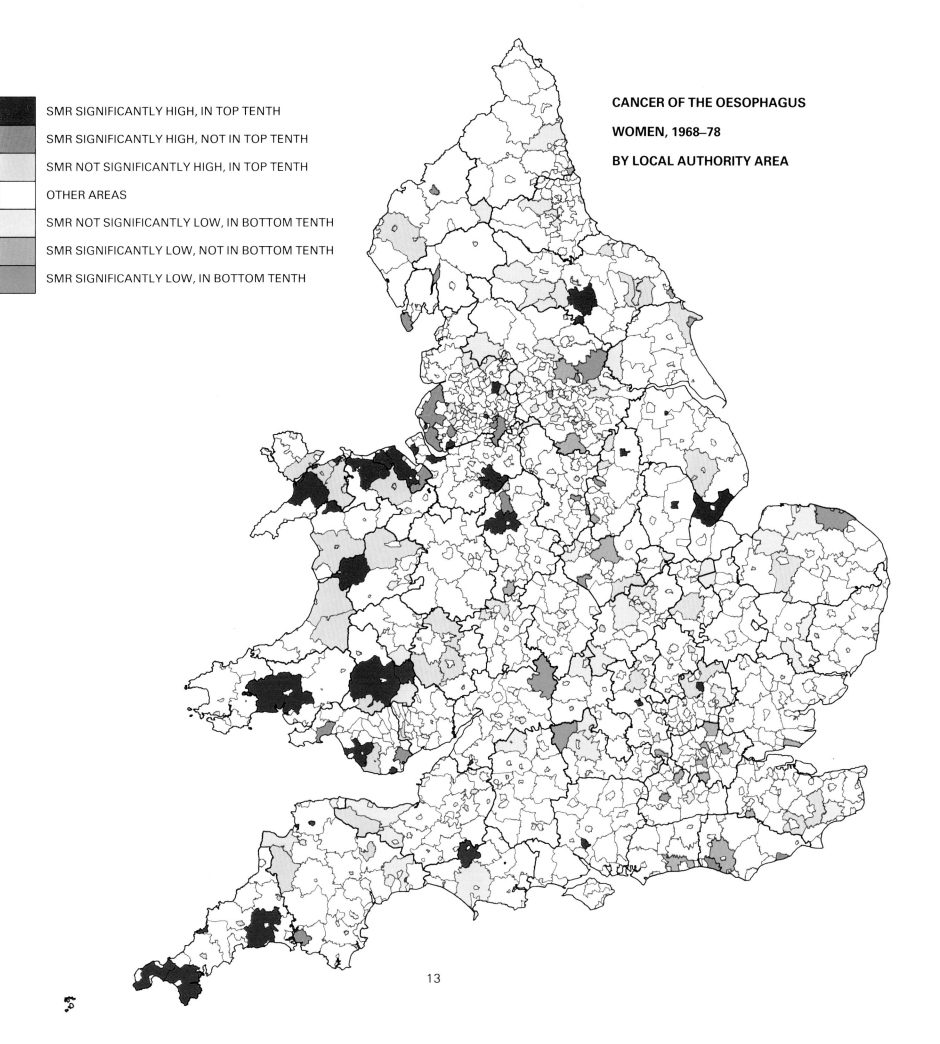

SMR SIGNIFICANTLY HIGH, IN TOP TENTH

SMR SIGNIFICANTLY HIGH, NOT IN TOP TENTH

SMR NOT SIGNIFICANTLY HIGH, IN TOP TENTH

OTHER AREAS

SMR NOT SIGNIFICANTLY LOW, IN BOTTOM TENTH

SMR SIGNIFICANTLY LOW, NOT IN BOTTOM TENTH

SMR SIGNIFICANTLY LOW, IN BOTTOM TENTH

CANCER OF THE OESOPHAGUS

WOMEN, 1968–78

BY LOCAL AUTHORITY AREA

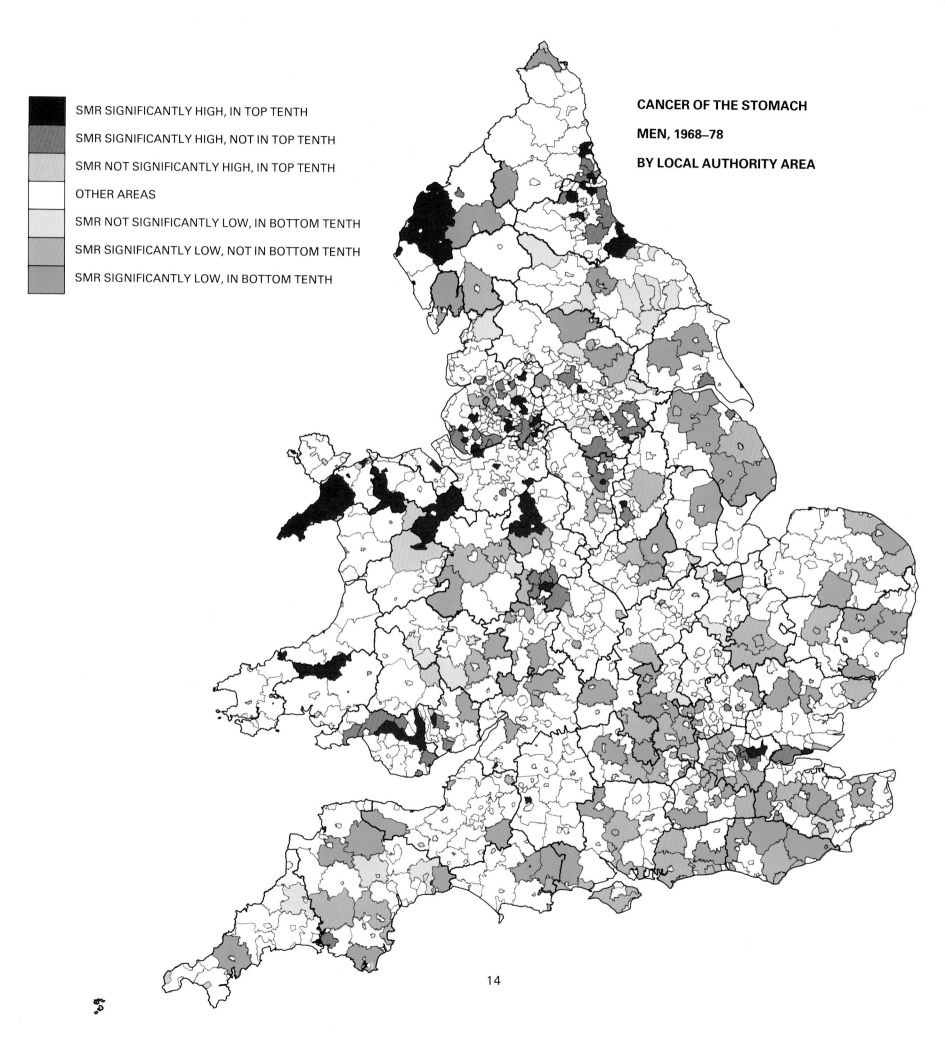

SMR SIGNIFICANTLY HIGH, IN TOP TENTH

SMR SIGNIFICANTLY HIGH, NOT IN TOP TENTH

SMR NOT SIGNIFICANTLY HIGH, IN TOP TENTH

OTHER AREAS

SMR NOT SIGNIFICANTLY LOW, IN BOTTOM TENTH

SMR SIGNIFICANTLY LOW, NOT IN BOTTOM TENTH

SMR SIGNIFICANTLY LOW, IN BOTTOM TENTH

CANCER OF THE STOMACH

MEN, 1968–78

BY LOCAL AUTHORITY AREA

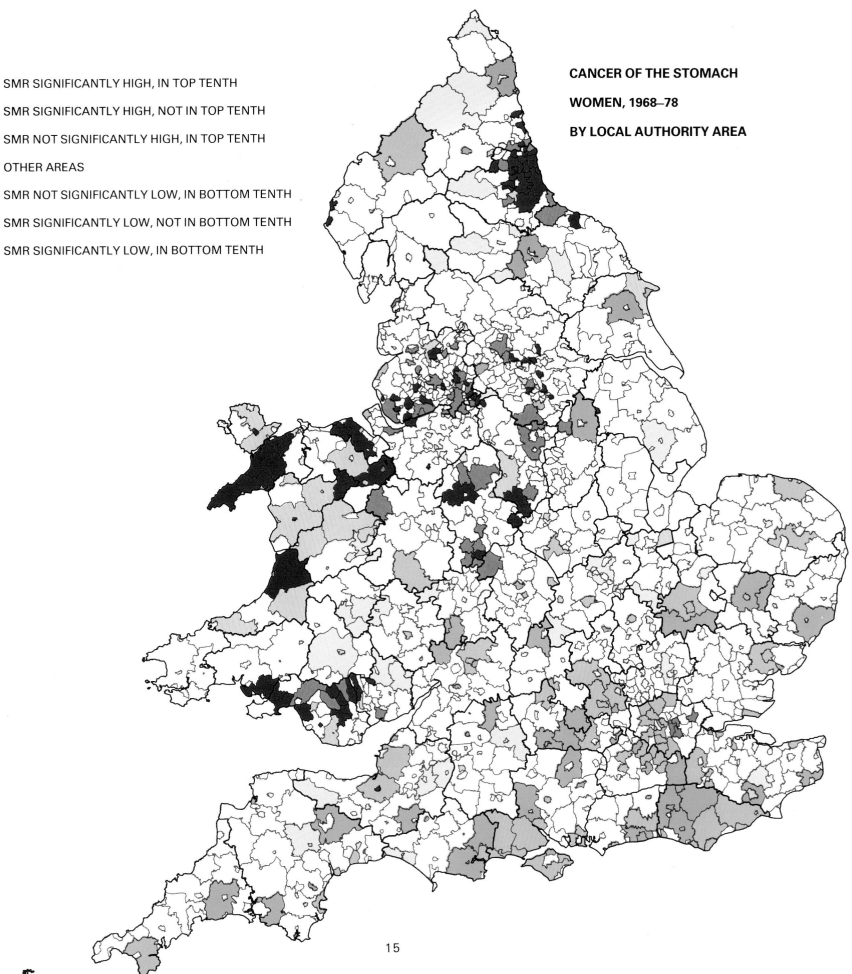

SMR SIGNIFICANTLY HIGH, IN TOP TENTH

SMR SIGNIFICANTLY HIGH, NOT IN TOP TENTH

SMR NOT SIGNIFICANTLY HIGH, IN TOP TENTH

OTHER AREAS

SMR NOT SIGNIFICANTLY LOW, IN BOTTOM TENTH

SMR SIGNIFICANTLY LOW, NOT IN BOTTOM TENTH

SMR SIGNIFICANTLY LOW, IN BOTTOM TENTH

CANCER OF THE STOMACH

WOMEN, 1968–78

BY LOCAL AUTHORITY AREA

15

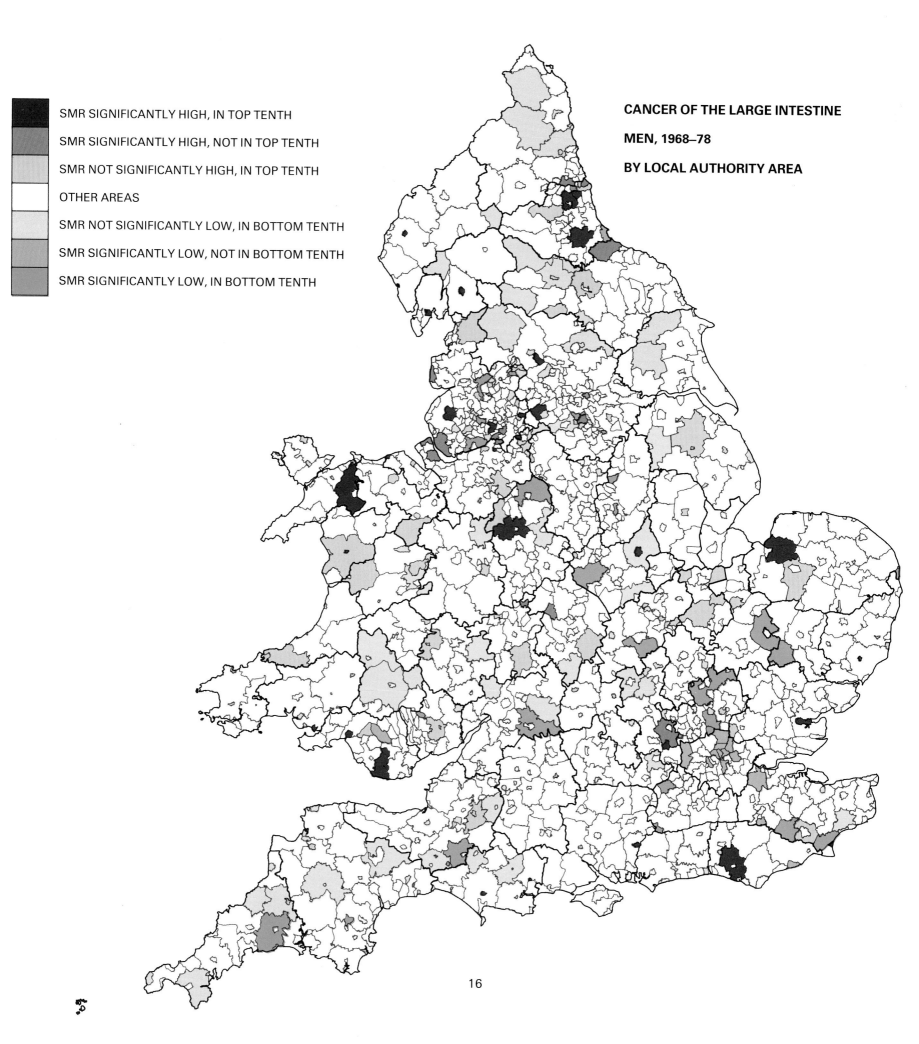

SMR SIGNIFICANTLY HIGH, IN TOP TENTH

SMR SIGNIFICANTLY HIGH, NOT IN TOP TENTH

SMR NOT SIGNIFICANTLY HIGH, IN TOP TENTH

OTHER AREAS

SMR NOT SIGNIFICANTLY LOW, IN BOTTOM TENTH

SMR SIGNIFICANTLY LOW, NOT IN BOTTOM TENTH

SMR SIGNIFICANTLY LOW, IN BOTTOM TENTH

CANCER OF THE LARGE INTESTINE

MEN, 1968–78

BY LOCAL AUTHORITY AREA

16

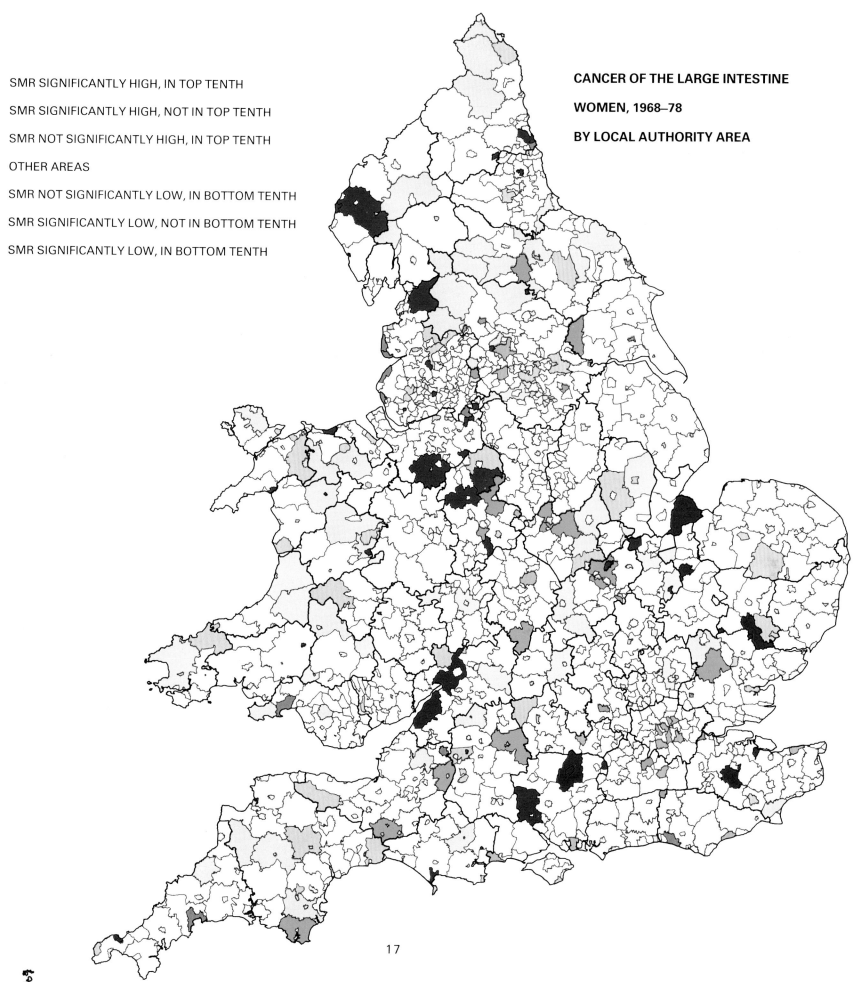

SMR SIGNIFICANTLY HIGH, IN TOP TENTH

SMR SIGNIFICANTLY HIGH, NOT IN TOP TENTH

SMR NOT SIGNIFICANTLY HIGH, IN TOP TENTH

OTHER AREAS

SMR NOT SIGNIFICANTLY LOW, IN BOTTOM TENTH

SMR SIGNIFICANTLY LOW, NOT IN BOTTOM TENTH

SMR SIGNIFICANTLY LOW, IN BOTTOM TENTH

CANCER OF THE LARGE INTESTINE

WOMEN, 1968–78

BY LOCAL AUTHORITY AREA

17

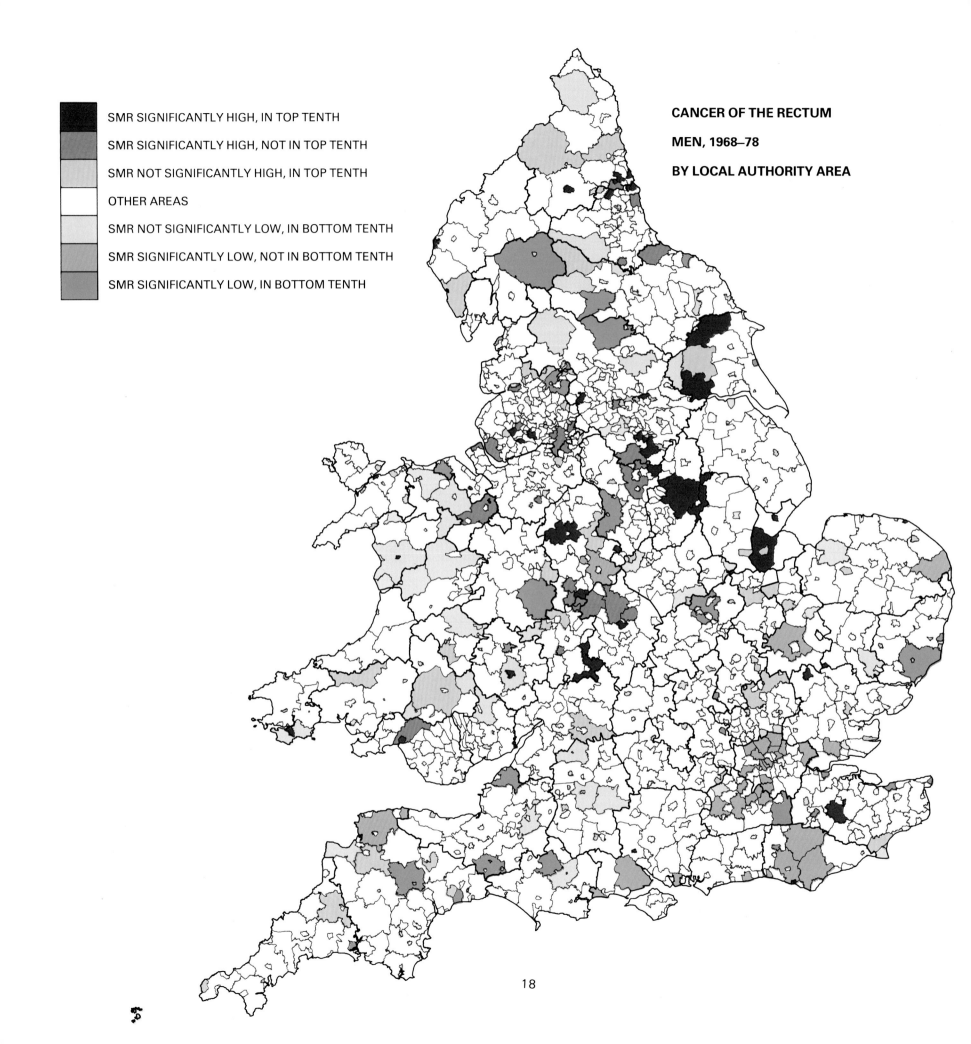

SMR SIGNIFICANTLY HIGH, IN TOP TENTH

SMR SIGNIFICANTLY HIGH, NOT IN TOP TENTH

SMR NOT SIGNIFICANTLY HIGH, IN TOP TENTH

OTHER AREAS

SMR NOT SIGNIFICANTLY LOW, IN BOTTOM TENTH

SMR SIGNIFICANTLY LOW, NOT IN BOTTOM TENTH

SMR SIGNIFICANTLY LOW, IN BOTTOM TENTH

CANCER OF THE RECTUM

MEN, 1968–78

BY LOCAL AUTHORITY AREA

18

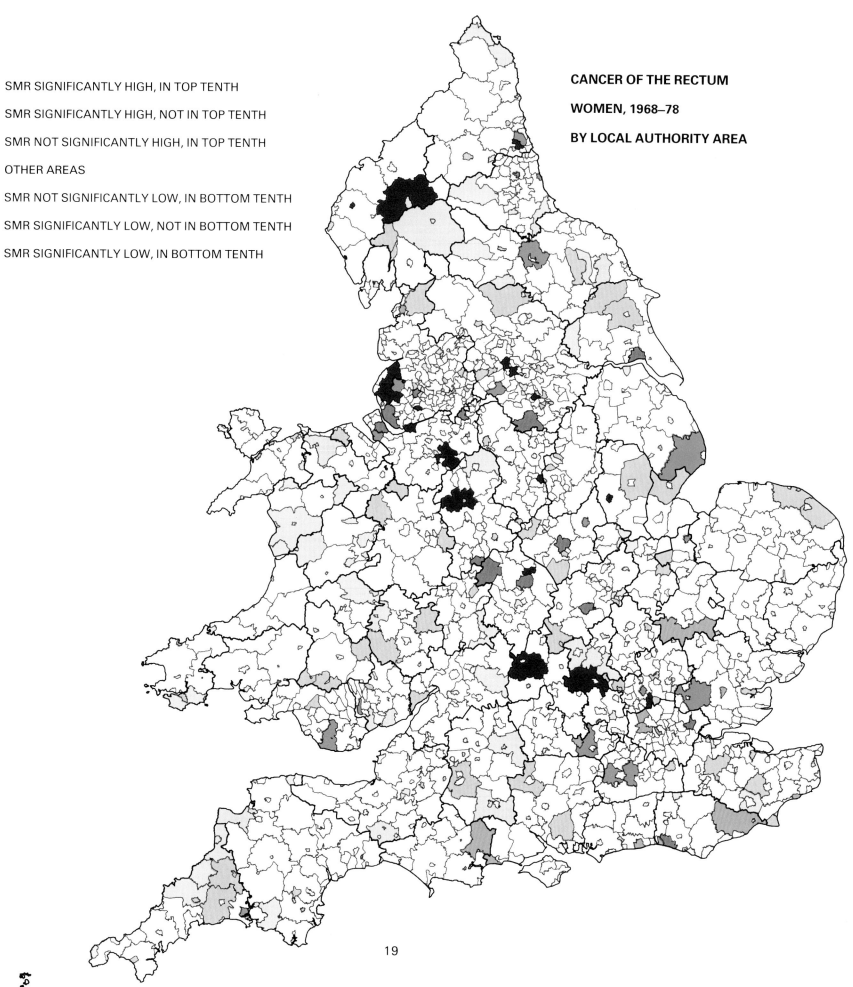

SMR SIGNIFICANTLY HIGH, IN TOP TENTH

SMR SIGNIFICANTLY HIGH, NOT IN TOP TENTH

SMR NOT SIGNIFICANTLY HIGH, IN TOP TENTH

OTHER AREAS

SMR NOT SIGNIFICANTLY LOW, IN BOTTOM TENTH

SMR SIGNIFICANTLY LOW, NOT IN BOTTOM TENTH

SMR SIGNIFICANTLY LOW, IN BOTTOM TENTH

CANCER OF THE RECTUM

WOMEN, 1968–78

BY LOCAL AUTHORITY AREA

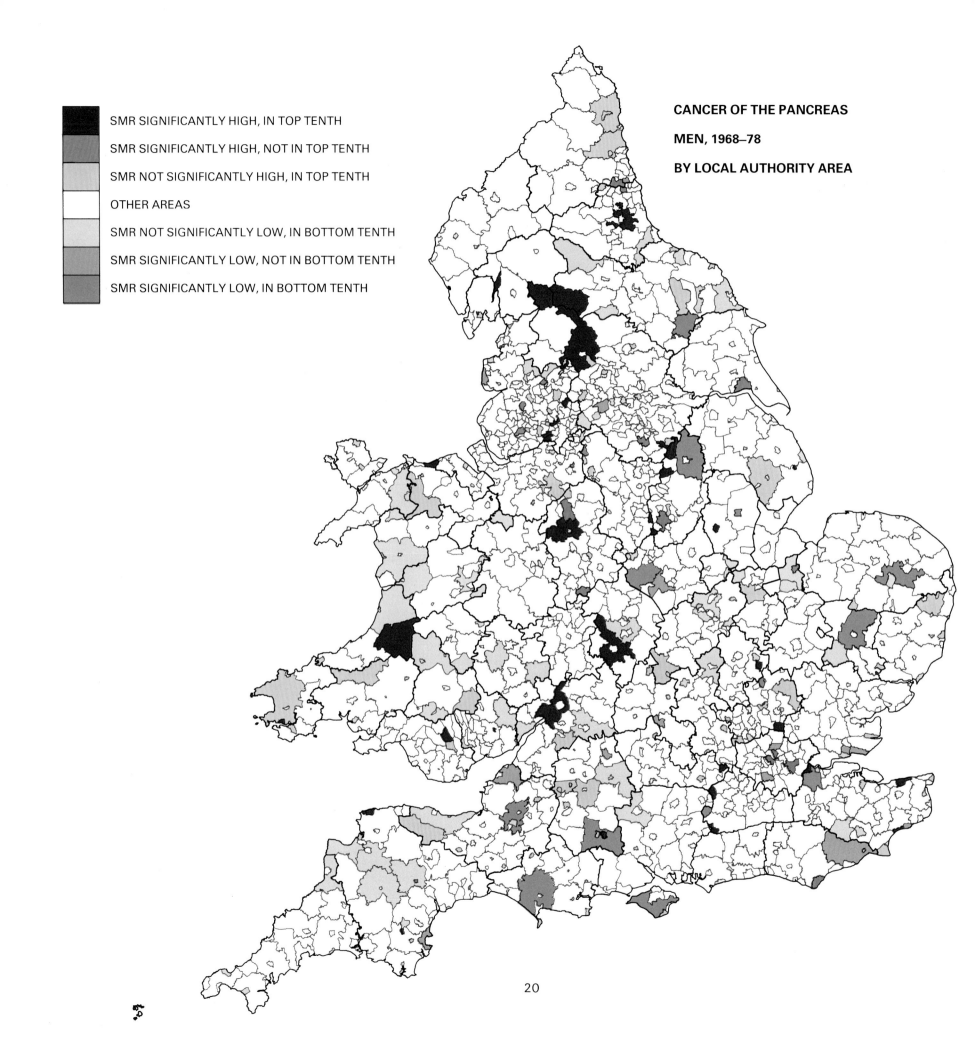

SMR SIGNIFICANTLY HIGH, IN TOP TENTH

SMR SIGNIFICANTLY HIGH, NOT IN TOP TENTH

SMR NOT SIGNIFICANTLY HIGH, IN TOP TENTH

OTHER AREAS

SMR NOT SIGNIFICANTLY LOW, IN BOTTOM TENTH

SMR SIGNIFICANTLY LOW, NOT IN BOTTOM TENTH

SMR SIGNIFICANTLY LOW, IN BOTTOM TENTH

CANCER OF THE PANCREAS

MEN, 1968–78

BY LOCAL AUTHORITY AREA

20

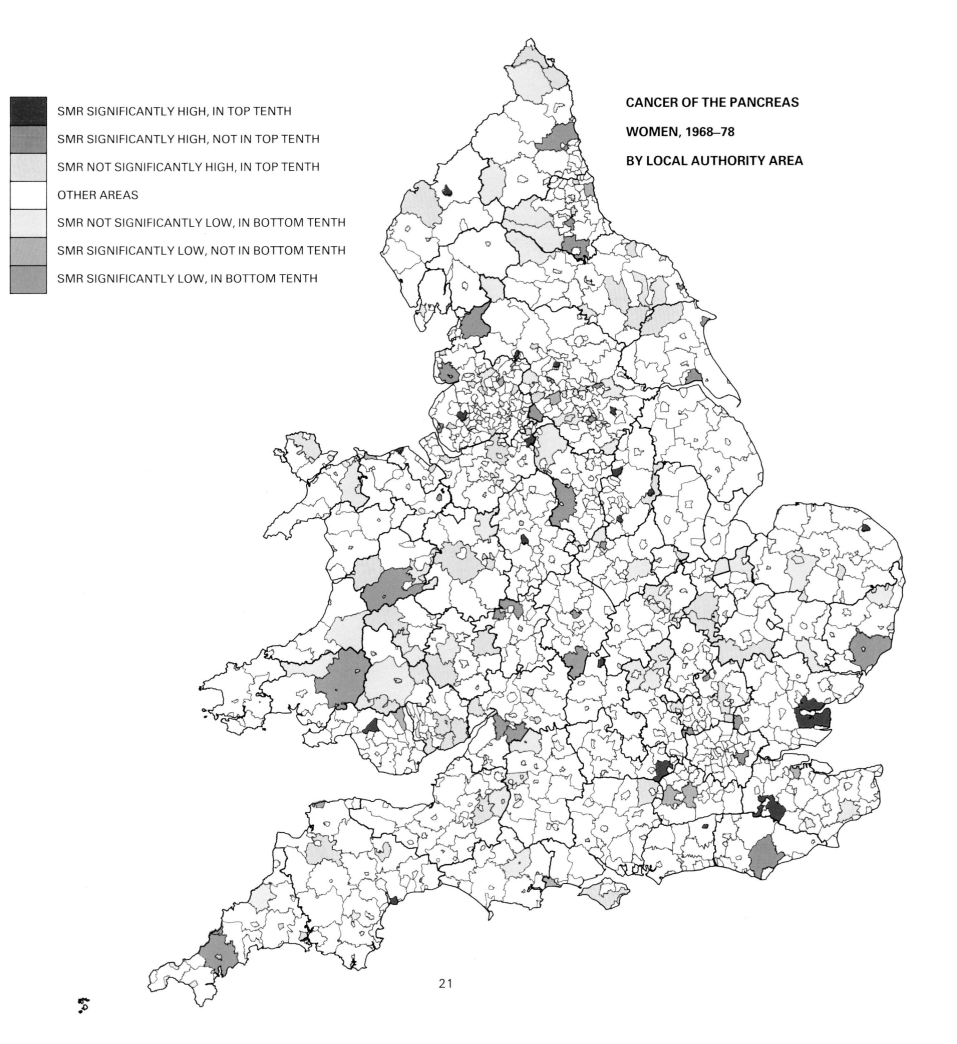

SMR SIGNIFICANTLY HIGH, IN TOP TENTH

SMR SIGNIFICANTLY HIGH, NOT IN TOP TENTH

SMR NOT SIGNIFICANTLY HIGH, IN TOP TENTH

OTHER AREAS

SMR NOT SIGNIFICANTLY LOW, IN BOTTOM TENTH

SMR SIGNIFICANTLY LOW, NOT IN BOTTOM TENTH

SMR SIGNIFICANTLY LOW, IN BOTTOM TENTH

CANCER OF THE PANCREAS

WOMEN, 1968–78

BY LOCAL AUTHORITY AREA

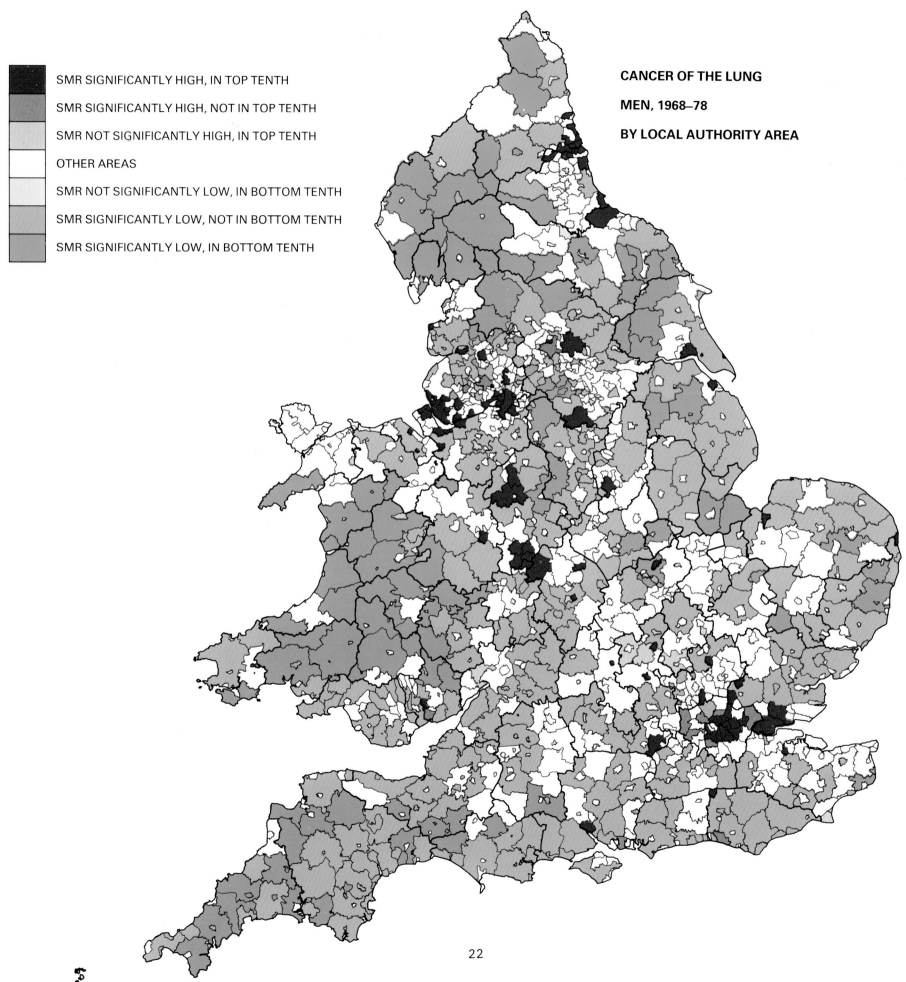

SMR SIGNIFICANTLY HIGH, IN TOP TENTH

SMR SIGNIFICANTLY HIGH, NOT IN TOP TENTH

SMR NOT SIGNIFICANTLY HIGH, IN TOP TENTH

OTHER AREAS

SMR NOT SIGNIFICANTLY LOW, IN BOTTOM TENTH

SMR SIGNIFICANTLY LOW, NOT IN BOTTOM TENTH

SMR SIGNIFICANTLY LOW, IN BOTTOM TENTH

CANCER OF THE LUNG

MEN, 1968–78

BY LOCAL AUTHORITY AREA

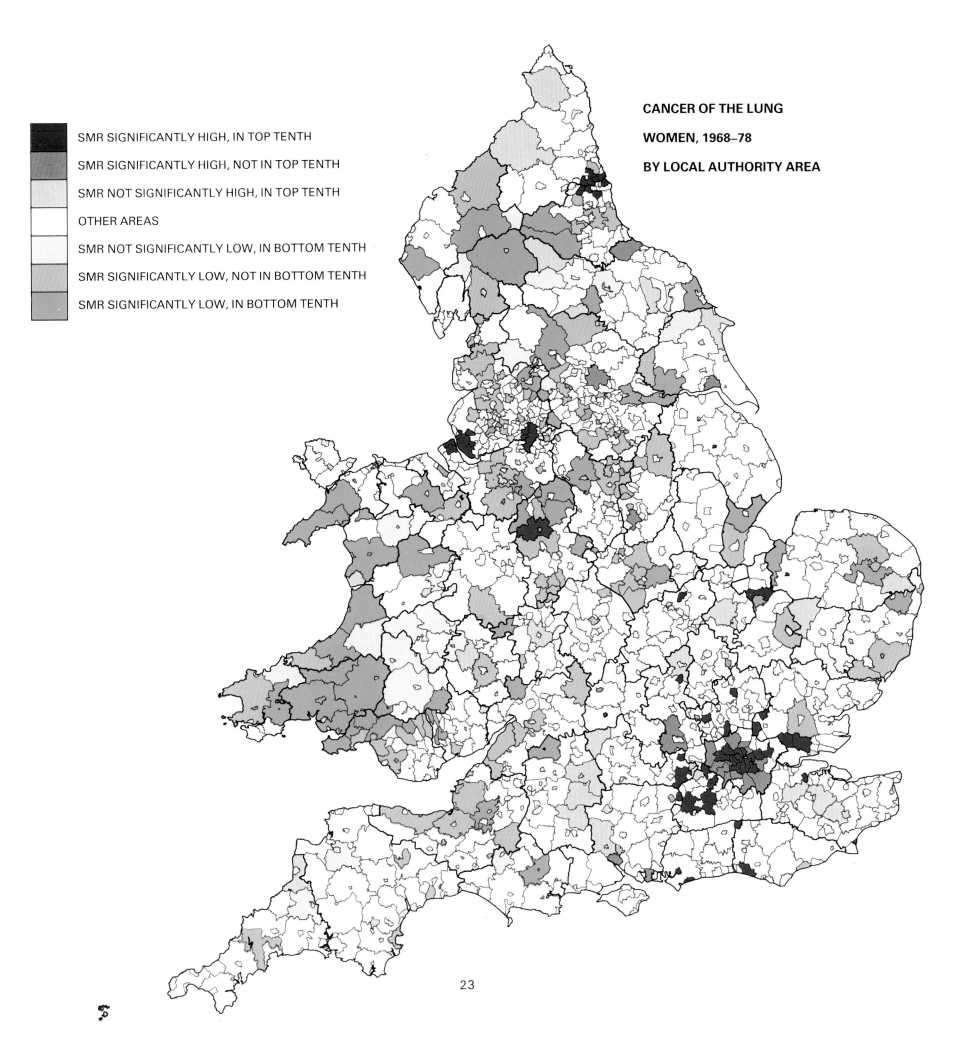

SMR SIGNIFICANTLY HIGH, IN TOP TENTH

SMR SIGNIFICANTLY HIGH, NOT IN TOP TENTH

SMR NOT SIGNIFICANTLY HIGH, IN TOP TENTH

OTHER AREAS

SMR NOT SIGNIFICANTLY LOW, IN BOTTOM TENTH

SMR SIGNIFICANTLY LOW, NOT IN BOTTOM TENTH

SMR SIGNIFICANTLY LOW, IN BOTTOM TENTH

CANCER OF THE LUNG

WOMEN, 1968–78

BY LOCAL AUTHORITY AREA

23

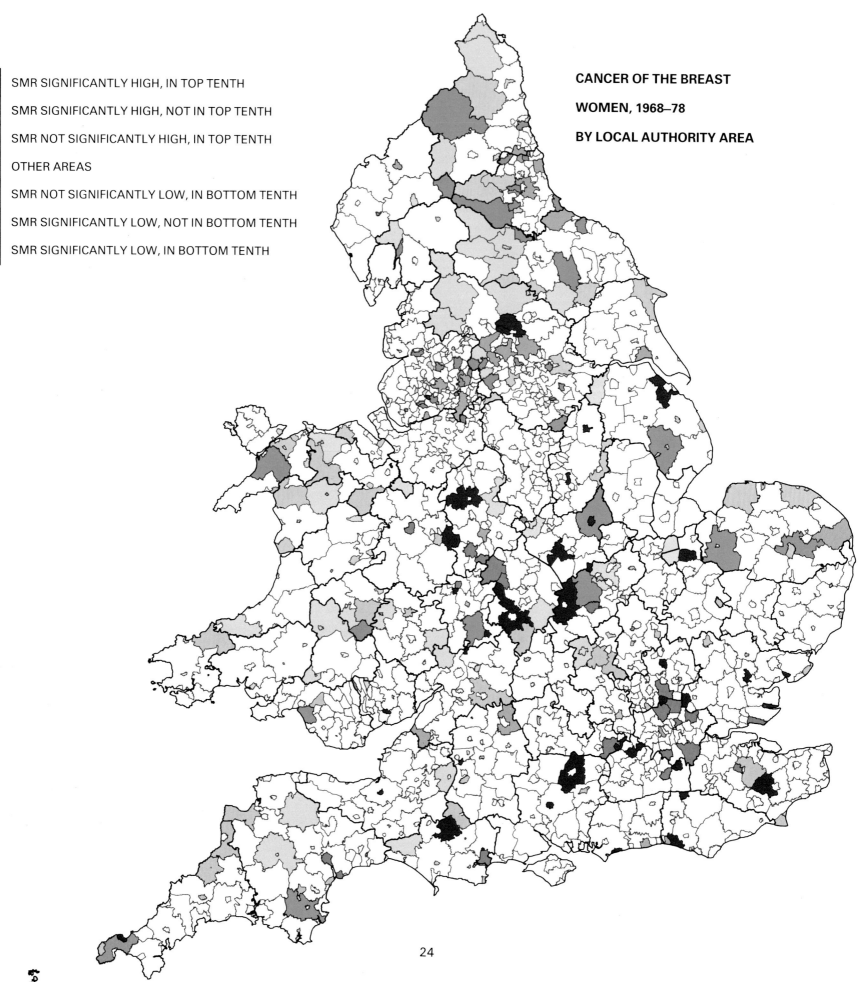

SMR SIGNIFICANTLY HIGH, IN TOP TENTH

SMR SIGNIFICANTLY HIGH, NOT IN TOP TENTH

SMR NOT SIGNIFICANTLY HIGH, IN TOP TENTH

OTHER AREAS

SMR NOT SIGNIFICANTLY LOW, IN BOTTOM TENTH

SMR SIGNIFICANTLY LOW, NOT IN BOTTOM TENTH

SMR SIGNIFICANTLY LOW, IN BOTTOM TENTH

CANCER OF THE BREAST

WOMEN, 1968–78

BY LOCAL AUTHORITY AREA

24

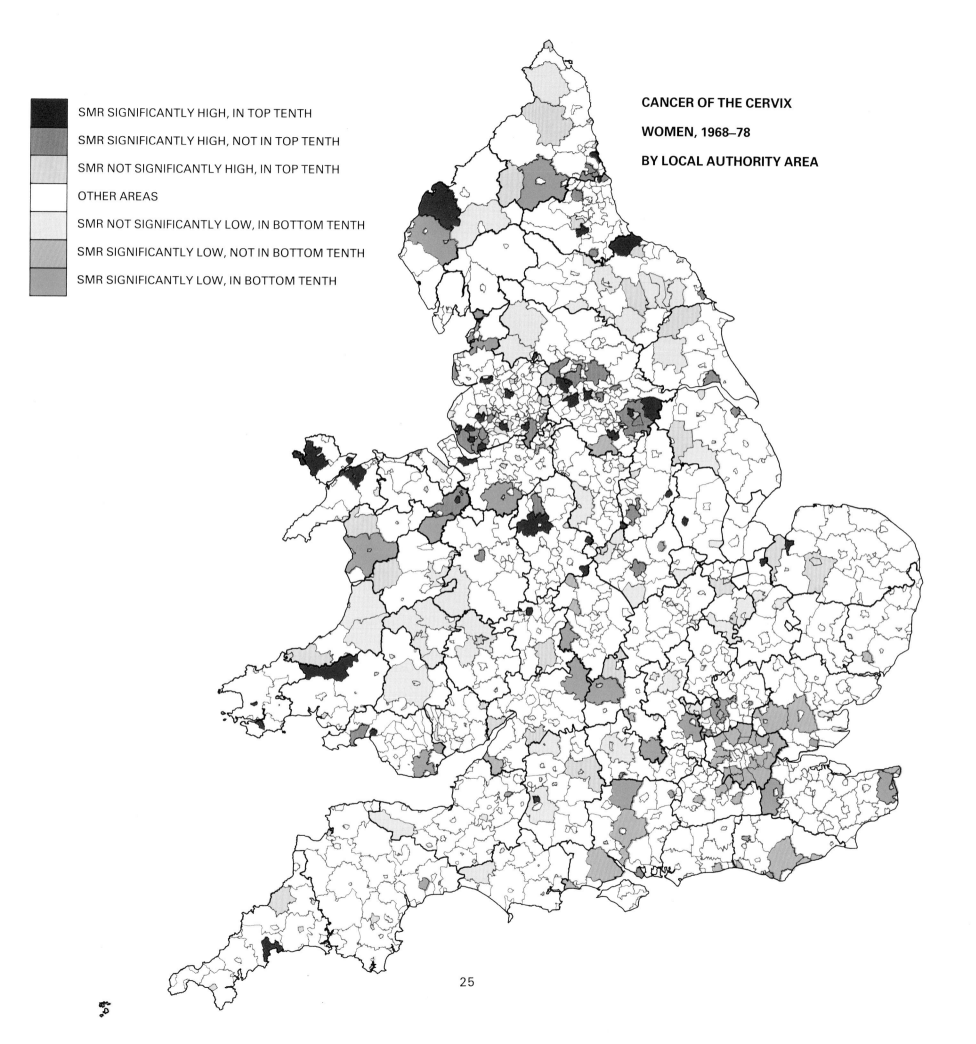

CANCER OF THE CERVIX

WOMEN, 1968–78

BY LOCAL AUTHORITY AREA

SMR SIGNIFICANTLY HIGH, IN TOP TENTH

SMR SIGNIFICANTLY HIGH, NOT IN TOP TENTH

SMR NOT SIGNIFICANTLY HIGH, IN TOP TENTH

OTHER AREAS

SMR NOT SIGNIFICANTLY LOW, IN BOTTOM TENTH

SMR SIGNIFICANTLY LOW, NOT IN BOTTOM TENTH

SMR SIGNIFICANTLY LOW, IN BOTTOM TENTH

25

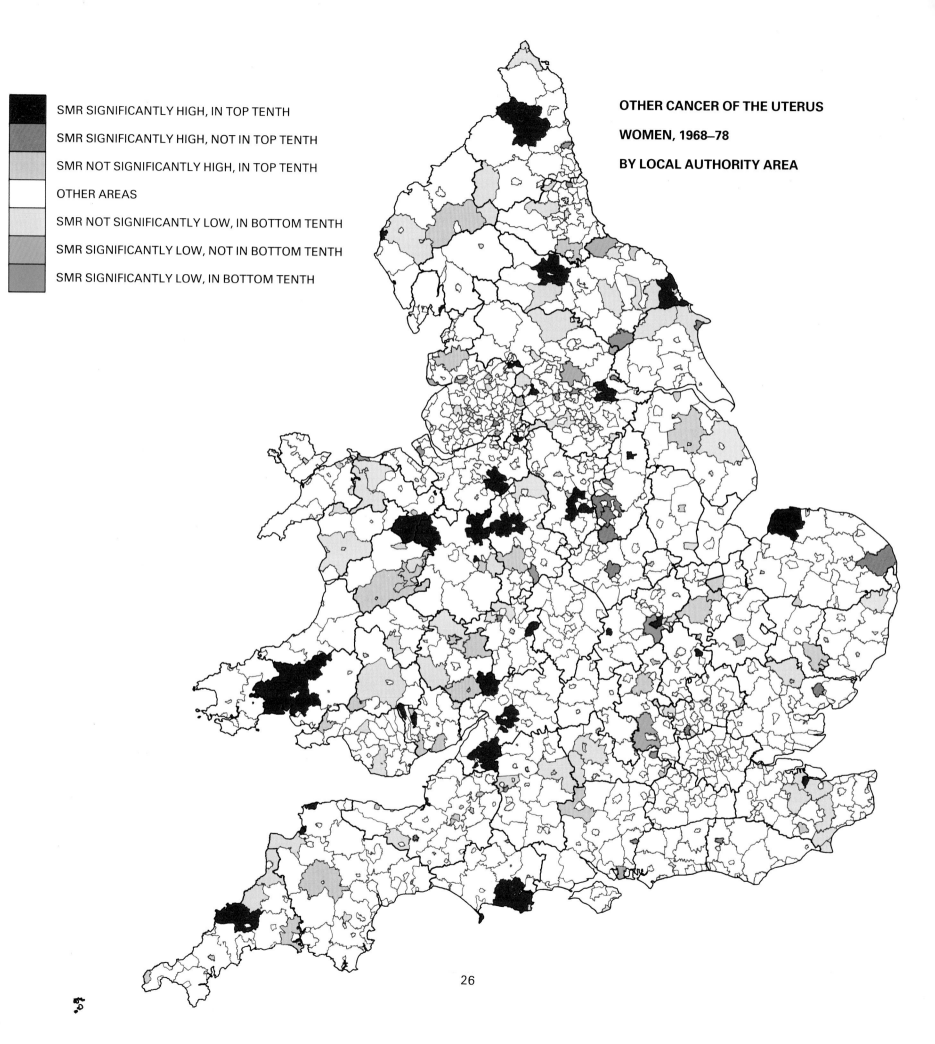

SMR SIGNIFICANTLY HIGH, IN TOP TENTH

SMR SIGNIFICANTLY HIGH, NOT IN TOP TENTH

SMR NOT SIGNIFICANTLY HIGH, IN TOP TENTH

OTHER AREAS

SMR NOT SIGNIFICANTLY LOW, IN BOTTOM TENTH

SMR SIGNIFICANTLY LOW, NOT IN BOTTOM TENTH

SMR SIGNIFICANTLY LOW, IN BOTTOM TENTH

OTHER CANCER OF THE UTERUS

WOMEN, 1968–78

BY LOCAL AUTHORITY AREA

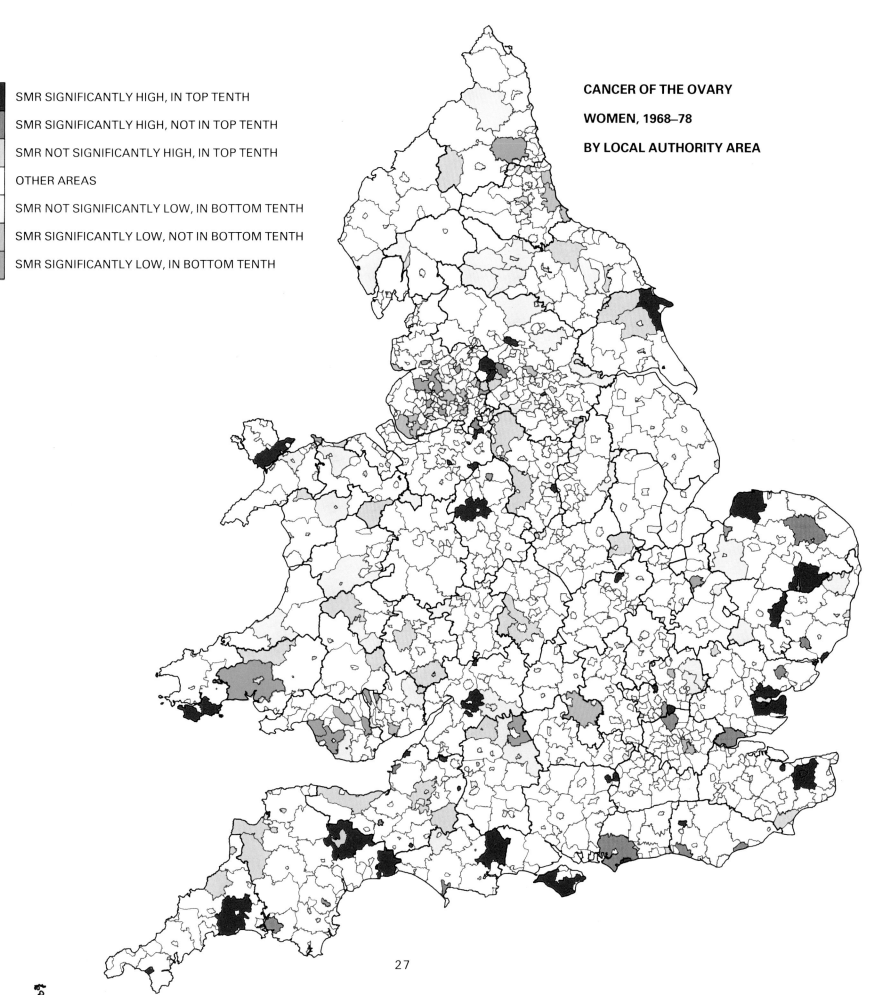

SMR SIGNIFICANTLY HIGH, IN TOP TENTH

SMR SIGNIFICANTLY HIGH, NOT IN TOP TENTH

SMR NOT SIGNIFICANTLY HIGH, IN TOP TENTH

OTHER AREAS

SMR NOT SIGNIFICANTLY LOW, IN BOTTOM TENTH

SMR SIGNIFICANTLY LOW, NOT IN BOTTOM TENTH

SMR SIGNIFICANTLY LOW, IN BOTTOM TENTH

CANCER OF THE OVARY

WOMEN, 1968–78

BY LOCAL AUTHORITY AREA

27

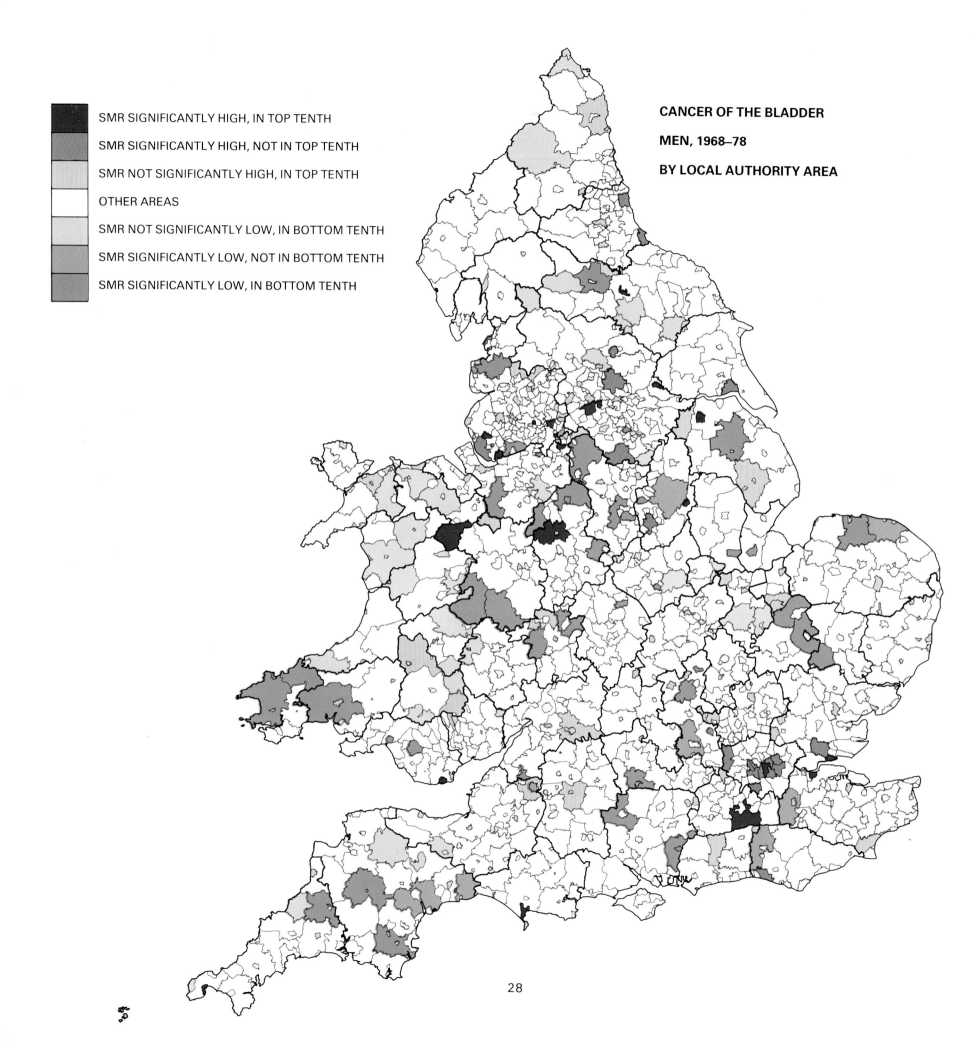

SMR SIGNIFICANTLY HIGH, IN TOP TENTH

SMR SIGNIFICANTLY HIGH, NOT IN TOP TENTH

SMR NOT SIGNIFICANTLY HIGH, IN TOP TENTH

OTHER AREAS

SMR NOT SIGNIFICANTLY LOW, IN BOTTOM TENTH

SMR SIGNIFICANTLY LOW, NOT IN BOTTOM TENTH

SMR SIGNIFICANTLY LOW, IN BOTTOM TENTH

CANCER OF THE BLADDER

MEN, 1968–78

BY LOCAL AUTHORITY AREA

28

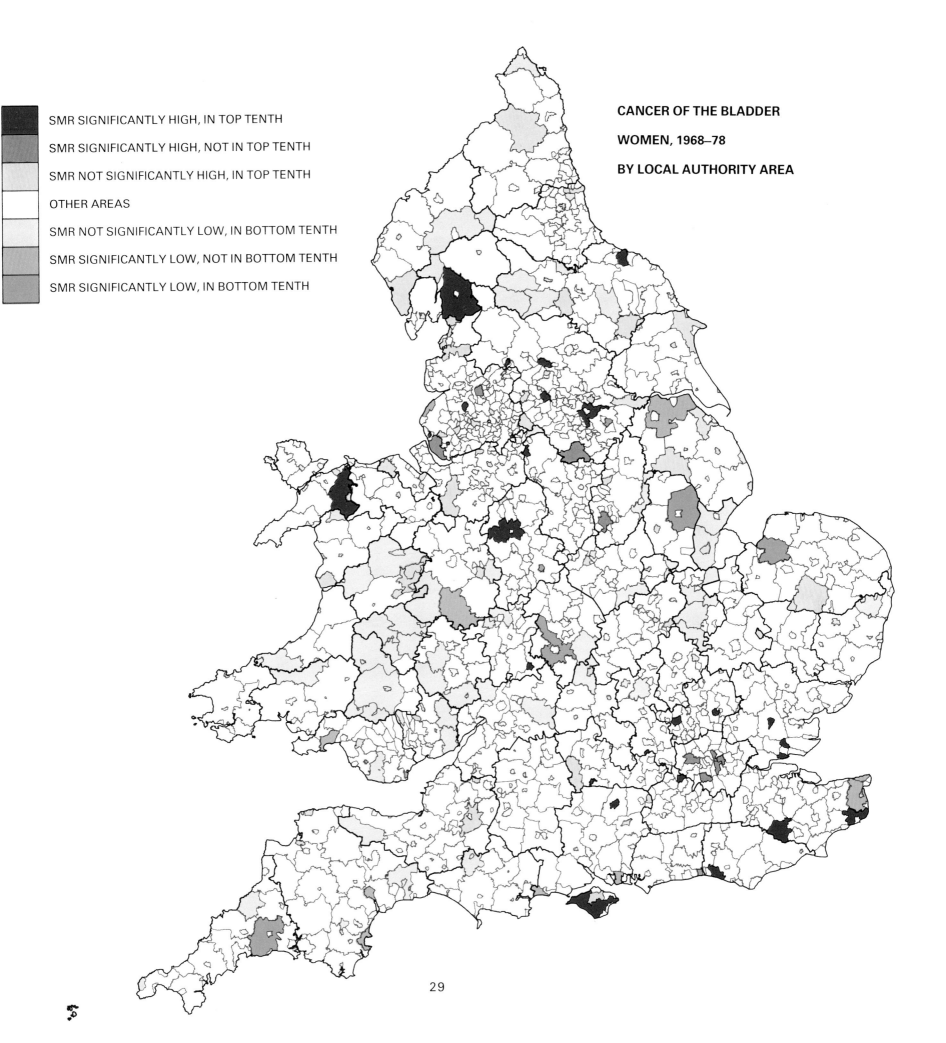

SMR SIGNIFICANTLY HIGH, IN TOP TENTH

SMR SIGNIFICANTLY HIGH, NOT IN TOP TENTH

SMR NOT SIGNIFICANTLY HIGH, IN TOP TENTH

OTHER AREAS

SMR NOT SIGNIFICANTLY LOW, IN BOTTOM TENTH

SMR SIGNIFICANTLY LOW, NOT IN BOTTOM TENTH

SMR SIGNIFICANTLY LOW, IN BOTTOM TENTH

CANCER OF THE BLADDER

WOMEN, 1968–78

BY LOCAL AUTHORITY AREA

29

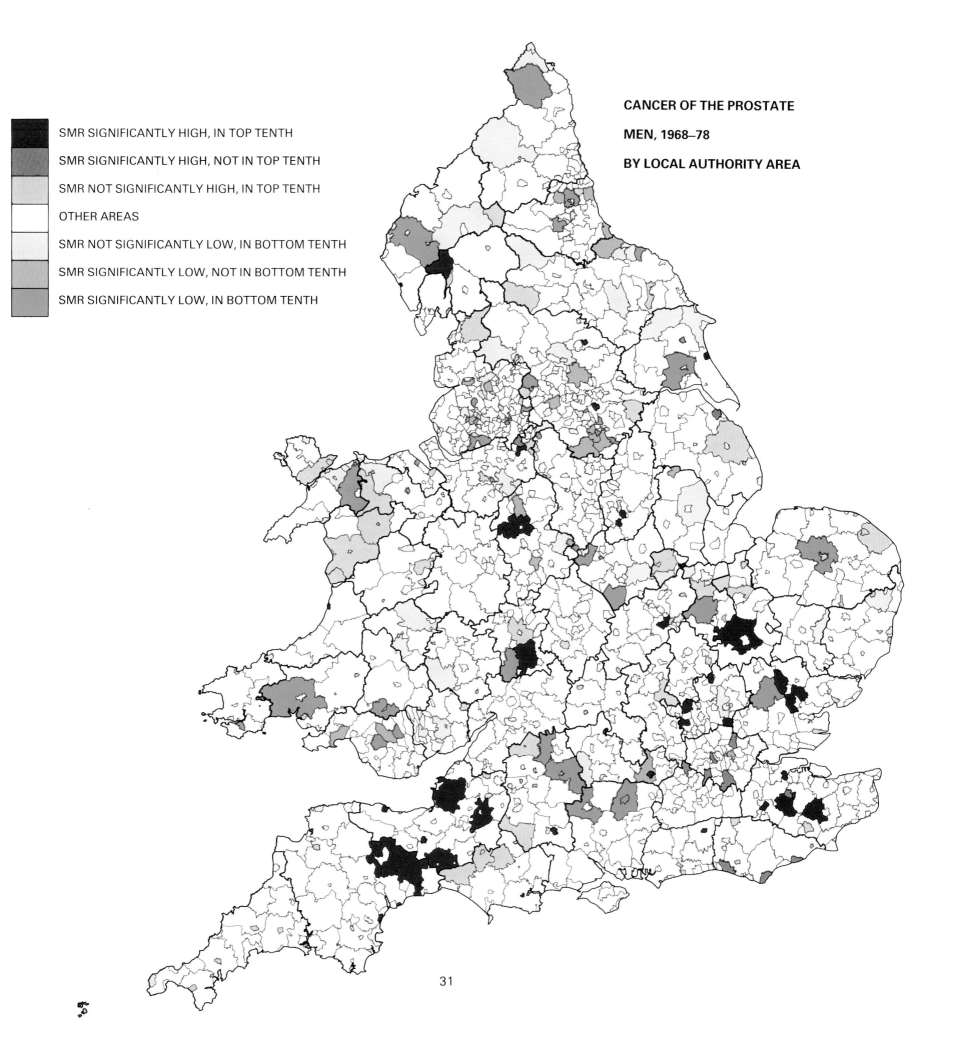

CANCER OF THE PROSTATE

MEN, 1968–78

BY LOCAL AUTHORITY AREA

SMR SIGNIFICANTLY HIGH, IN TOP TENTH

SMR SIGNIFICANTLY HIGH, NOT IN TOP TENTH

SMR NOT SIGNIFICANTLY HIGH, IN TOP TENTH

OTHER AREAS

SMR NOT SIGNIFICANTLY LOW, IN BOTTOM TENTH

SMR SIGNIFICANTLY LOW, NOT IN BOTTOM TENTH

SMR SIGNIFICANTLY LOW, IN BOTTOM TENTH

31

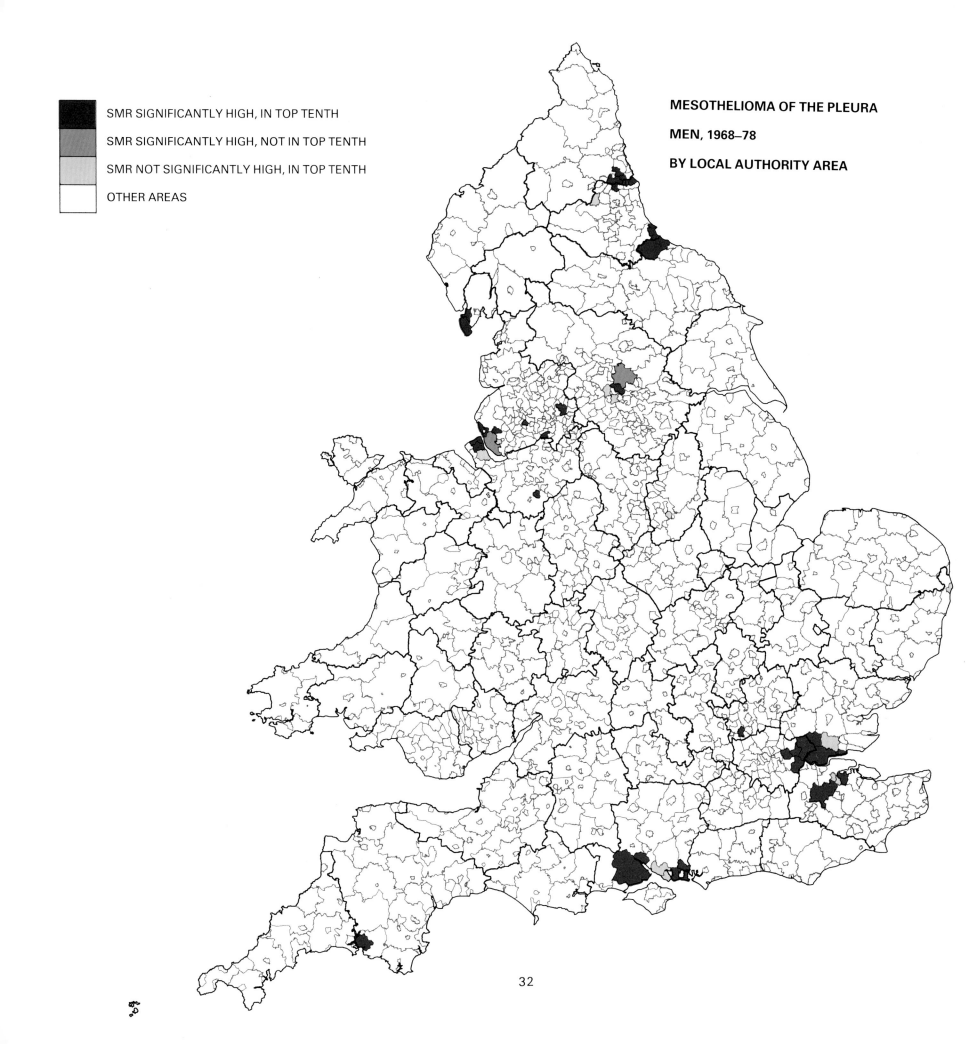

SMR SIGNIFICANTLY HIGH, IN TOP TENTH

SMR SIGNIFICANTLY HIGH, NOT IN TOP TENTH

SMR NOT SIGNIFICANTLY HIGH, IN TOP TENTH

OTHER AREAS

MESOTHELIOMA OF THE PLEURA

MEN, 1968–78

BY LOCAL AUTHORITY AREA

32

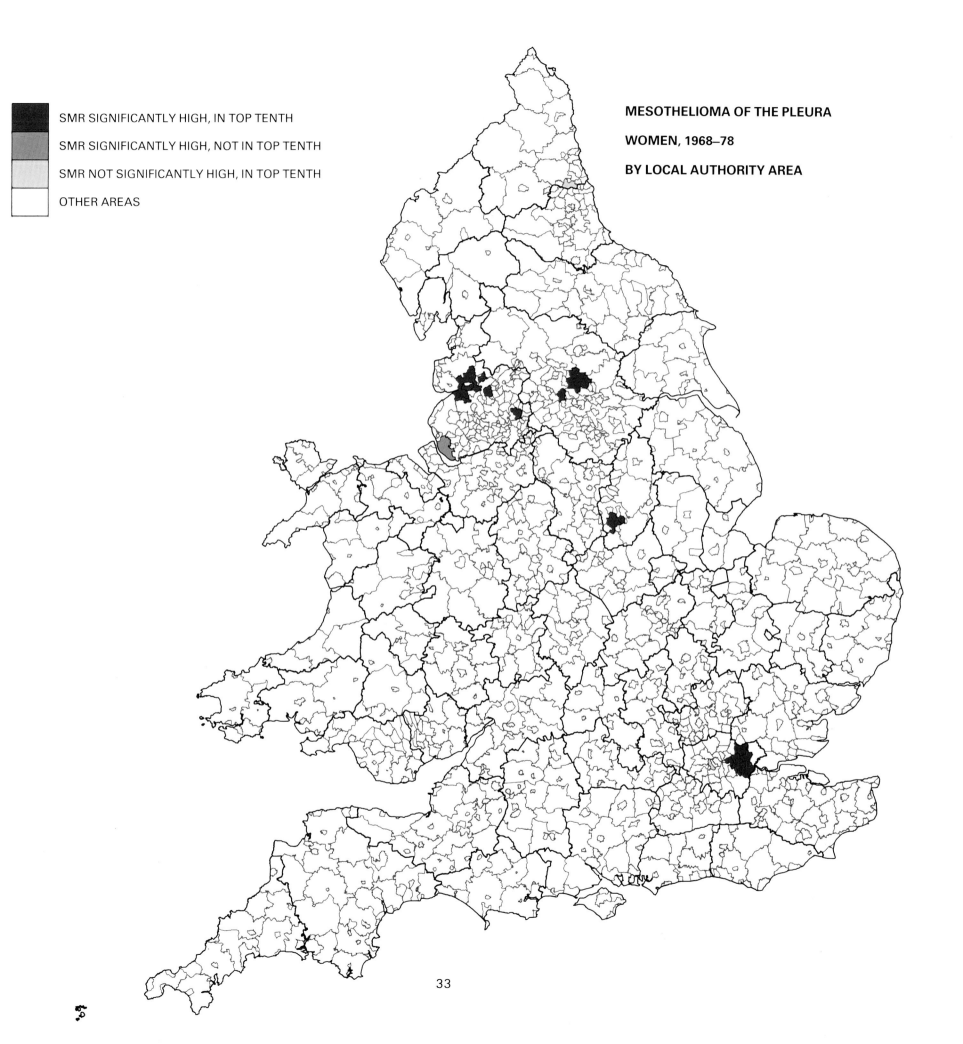

SMR SIGNIFICANTLY HIGH, IN TOP TENTH

SMR SIGNIFICANTLY HIGH, NOT IN TOP TENTH

SMR NOT SIGNIFICANTLY HIGH, IN TOP TENTH

OTHER AREAS

MESOTHELIOMA OF THE PLEURA

WOMEN, 1968–78

BY LOCAL AUTHORITY AREA

33

MORTALITY FROM ALL CAUSES OF DEATH
IN ENGLAND AND WALES DURING 1968–78

NUMBER OF DEATHS DURING 1968–78 AND AVERAGE ANNUAL
DEATH RATES PER MILLION BY SEX AND AGE GROUPS

AGE GROUP (YEARS)	MEN		WOMEN	
	NUMBER OF DEATHS	RATE PER MILLION	NUMBER OF DEATHS	RATE PER MILLION
0	72,566	16,616	52,702	12,705
1–4	12,419	703	9,583	571
5–14	15,684	362	9,865	240
15–24	36,449	928	15,181	397
25–34	34,864	1,032	20,601	626
35–44	70,043	2,214	48,475	1,549
45–54	232,273	7,125	144,412	4,278
55–64	596,728	19,627	333,634	9,936
65–74	1,037,788	53,749	727,210	27,289
75+	1,134,131	139,990	1,801,824	103,587
ALL AGES	3,242,945	12,448	3,163,487	11,473

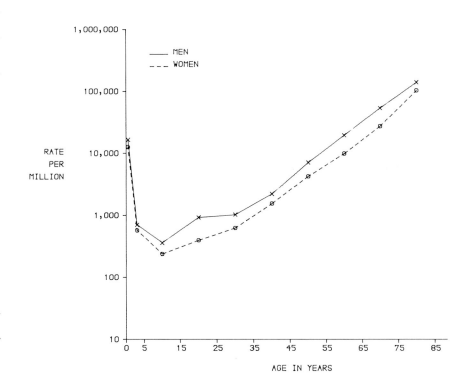

VALUES OF THE STANDARDISED MORTALITY RATIO
(SMR) WHICH DIVIDE THE 1366 LOCAL AUTHORITY
AREAS INTO TENTHS ACCORDING TO THE LEVEL
OF MORTALITY

PERCENTILE	STANDARDISED MORTALITY RATIO	
	MEN	WOMEN
10th	83.5	85.4
20th	88.0	89.5
30th	91.3	93.4
40th	94.8	96.8
50th	98.0	99.6
60th	101.5	103.0
70th	105.2	106.8
80th	109.4	111.4
90th	115.9	118.5
LOWEST SMR	57.9	50.7
HIGHEST SMR	179.1	215.1
NUMBER OF AREAS WITH ZERO DEATHS	0	0

NUMBER OF LOCAL AUTHORITY AREAS SHOWN ON MAP BY CATEGORY –
BASED ON STANDARDISED MORTALITY RATIO (SMR) DURING 1968–78

CATEGORY	NUMBER OF AREAS	
	MEN	WOMEN
SMR SIGNIFICANTLY HIGH, IN TOP TENTH	136	136
SMR SIGNIFICANTLY HIGH, NOT IN TOP TENTH	241	307
SMR NOT SIGNIFICANTLY HIGH, IN TOP TENTH	1	1
SMR NOT SIGNIFICANTLY LOW, IN BOTTOM TENTH	0	3
SMR SIGNIFICANTLY LOW, NOT IN BOTTOM TENTH	386	304
SMR SIGNIFICANTLY LOW, IN BOTTOM TENTH	137	134

ANY AREA WITH A HIGH SMR, BUT WHERE LESS THAN 4 DEATHS OCCURRED IS
NOT MAPPED

MORTALITY FROM ALL CANCERS
IN ENGLAND AND WALES DURING 1968–78

NUMBER OF DEATHS DURING 1968–78 AND AVERAGE ANNUAL DEATH RATES PER MILLION BY SEX AND AGE GROUPS

AGE GROUP (YEARS)	MEN		WOMEN	
	NUMBER OF DEATHS	RATE PER MILLION	NUMBER OF DEATHS	RATE PER MILLION
0	222	51	177	43
1–4	1,401	79	1,075	64
5–14	2,852	66	1,991	49
15–24	3,645	93	2,422	63
25–34	6,165	182	5,782	176
35–44	15,188	480	20,603	658
45–54	61,077	1,873	67,355	1,995
55–64	174,894	5,753	128,371	3,823
65–74	266,204	13,787	177,587	6,664
75+	180,367	22,263	203,236	11,684
ALL AGES	·712,015	2,733	608,599	2,207

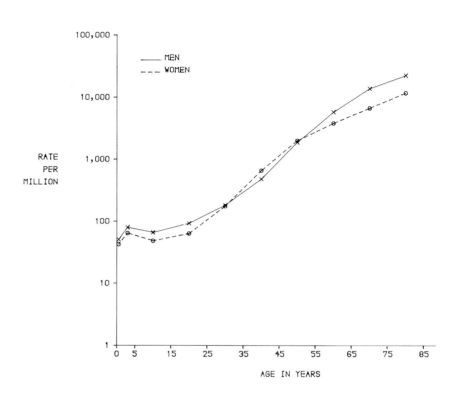

VALUES OF THE STANDARDISED MORTALITY RATIO (SMR) WHICH DIVIDE THE 1366 LOCAL AUTHORITY AREAS INTO TENTHS ACCORDING TO THE LEVEL OF MORTALITY

PERCENTILE	STANDARDISED MORTALITY RATIO	
	MEN	WOMEN
10th	78.6	85.8
20th	83.8	90.8
30th	87.4	93.6
40th	90.8	95.6
50th	93.6	97.9
60th	96.7	100.1
70th	99.8	102.4
80th	103.3	105.4
90th	110.2	110.9
LOWEST SMR	42.8	38.0
HIGHEST SMR	201.8	246.0
NUMBER OF AREAS WITH ZERO DEATHS	0	0

NUMBER OF LOCAL AUTHORITY AREAS SHOWN ON MAP BY CATEGORY – BASED ON STANDARDISED MORTALITY RATIO (SMR) DURING 1968–78

CATEGORY	NUMBER OF AREAS	
	MEN	WOMEN
SMR SIGNIFICANTLY HIGH, IN TOP TENTH	93	61
SMR SIGNIFICANTLY HIGH, NOT IN TOP TENTH	27	33
SMR NOT SIGNIFICANTLY HIGH, IN TOP TENTH	44	76
SMR NOT SIGNIFICANTLY LOW, IN BOTTOM TENTH	10	52
SMR SIGNIFICANTLY LOW, NOT IN BOTTOM TENTH	296	59
SMR SIGNIFICANTLY LOW, IN BOTTOM TENTH	127	85

ANY AREA WITH A HIGH SMR, BUT WHERE LESS THAN 4 DEATHS OCCURRED IS NOT MAPPED

MORTALITY FROM CANCER OF THE OESOPHAGUS
IN ENGLAND AND WALES DURING 1968–78

NUMBER OF DEATHS DURING 1968–78 AND AVERAGE ANNUAL DEATH RATES PER MILLION BY SEX AND AGE GROUPS

AGE GROUP (YEARS)	MEN		WOMEN	
	NUMBER OF DEATHS	RATE PER MILLION	NUMBER OF DEATHS	RATE PER MILLION
0	0	0.0	0	0.0
1–4	1	0.1	0	0.0
5–14	0	0.0	0	0.0
15–24	6	0.2	3	0.1
25–34	58	2	31	1
35–44	353	11	222	7
45–54	1,870	57	971	29
55–64	5,067	167	2,654	79
65–74	7,167	371	4,718	177
75+	5,472	675	7,083	407
ALL AGES	19,994	77	15,682	57

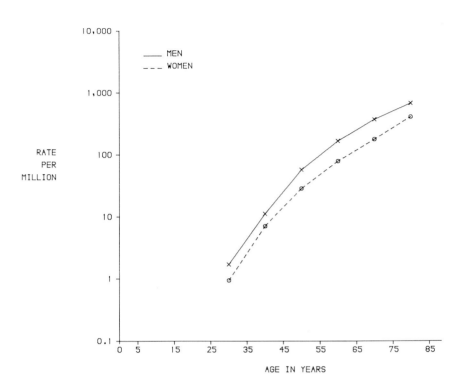

VALUES OF THE STANDARDISED MORTALITY RATIO (SMR) WHICH DIVIDE THE 1366 LOCAL AUTHORITY AREAS INTO TENTHS ACCORDING TO THE LEVEL OF MORTALITY

PERCENTILE	STANDARDISED MORTALITY RATIO	
	MEN	WOMEN
10th	46.8	43.0
20th	65.4	60.7
30th	79.0	76.2
40th	88.5	87.6
50th	96.2	97.7
60th	105.8	109.8
70th	116.8	123.1
80th	132.2	142.1
90th	159.2	174.6
LOWEST SMR	0.0	0.0
HIGHEST SMR	592.5	512.4
NUMBER OF AREAS WITH ZERO DEATHS	51	73

NUMBER OF LOCAL AUTHORITY AREAS SHOWN ON MAP BY CATEGORY – BASED ON STANDARDISED MORTALITY RATIO (SMR) DURING 1968–78

CATEGORY	NUMBER OF AREAS	
	MEN	WOMEN
SMR SIGNIFICANTLY HIGH, IN TOP TENTH	27	44
SMR SIGNIFICANTLY HIGH, NOT IN TOP TENTH	19	15
SMR NOT SIGNIFICANTLY HIGH, IN TOP TENTH	89	66
SMR NOT SIGNIFICANTLY LOW, IN BOTTOM TENTH	119	125
SMR SIGNIFICANTLY LOW, NOT IN BOTTOM TENTH	15	19
SMR SIGNIFICANTLY LOW, IN BOTTOM TENTH	18	12

ANY AREA WITH A HIGH SMR, BUT WHERE LESS THAN 4 DEATHS OCCURRED IS NOT MAPPED

MORTALITY FROM CANCER OF THE STOMACH
IN ENGLAND AND WALES DURING 1968–78

NUMBER OF DEATHS DURING 1968–78 AND AVERAGE ANNUAL DEATH RATES PER MILLION BY SEX AND AGE GROUPS

AGE GROUP (YEARS)	MEN		WOMEN	
	NUMBER OF DEATHS	RATE PER MILLION	NUMBER OF DEATHS	RATE PER MILLION
0	1	0.2	0	0.0
1–4	0	0.0	0	0.0
5–14	0	0.0	1	0.0
15–24	32	1	19	1
25–34	225	7	181	6
35–44	1,307	41	750	24
45–54	5,944	182	2,573	76
55–64	18,646	613	7,794	232
65–74	30,549	1,582	17,244	647
75+	20,917	2,582	27,787	1,597
ALL AGES	77,621	298	56,349	204

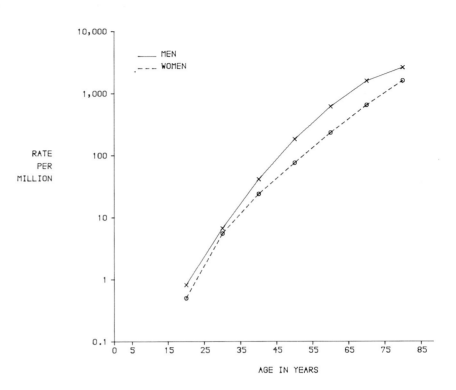

VALUES OF THE STANDARDISED MORTALITY RATIO (SMR) WHICH DIVIDE THE 1366 LOCAL AUTHORITY AREAS INTO TENTHS ACCORDING TO THE LEVEL OF MORTALITY

PERCENTILE	STANDARDISED MORTALITY RATIO	
	MEN	WOMEN
10th	63.3	58.0
20th	74.1	69.3
30th	81.0	77.3
40th	86.8	86.1
50th	94.7	93.5
60th	102.7	102.5
70th	112.1	111.8
80th	121.8	126.1
90th	135.6	143.0
LOWEST SMR	0.0	0.0
HIGHEST SMR	304.1	411.9
NUMBER OF AREAS WITH ZERO DEATHS	3	10

NUMBER OF LOCAL AUTHORITY AREAS SHOWN ON MAP BY CATEGORY – BASED ON STANDARDISED MORTALITY RATIO (SMR) DURING 1968–78

CATEGORY	NUMBER OF AREAS	
	MEN	WOMEN
SMR SIGNIFICANTLY HIGH, IN TOP TENTH	76	83
SMR SIGNIFICANTLY HIGH, NOT IN TOP TENTH	56	50
SMR NOT SIGNIFICANTLY HIGH, IN TOP TENTH	58	52
SMR NOT SIGNIFICANTLY LOW, IN BOTTOM TENTH	55	75
SMR SIGNIFICANTLY LOW, NOT IN BOTTOM TENTH	86	83
SMR SIGNIFICANTLY LOW, IN BOTTOM TENTH	82	62

ANY AREA WITH A HIGH SMR, BUT WHERE LESS THAN 4 DEATHS OCCURRED IS NOT MAPPED

MORTALITY FROM CANCER OF THE LARGE INTESTINE
IN ENGLAND AND WALES DURING 1968–78

NUMBER OF DEATHS DURING 1968–78 AND AVERAGE ANNUAL DEATH RATES PER MILLION BY SEX AND AGE GROUPS

AGE GROUP (YEARS)	MEN		WOMEN	
	NUMBER OF DEATHS	RATE PER MILLION	NUMBER OF DEATHS	RATE PER MILLION
0	0	0.0	0	0.0
1–4	0	0.0	0	0.0
5–14	8	0.2	4	0.1
15–24	38	1	34	1
25–34	291	9	234	7
35–44	1,183	37	1,159	37
45–54	3,713	114	4,065	120
55–64	9,568	315	10,847	323
65–74	16,521	856	19,545	733
75+	15,271	1,885	30,935	1,778
ALL AGES	46,593	179	66,823	242

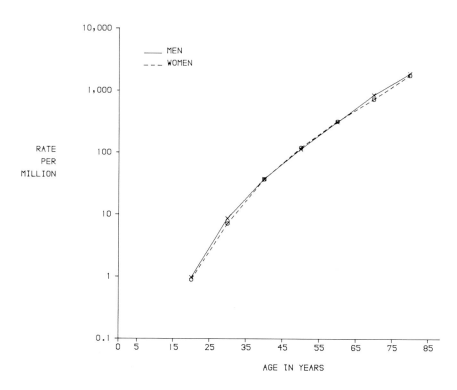

VALUES OF THE STANDARDISED MORTALITY RATIO (SMR) WHICH DIVIDE THE 1366 LOCAL AUTHORITY AREAS INTO TENTHS ACCORDING TO THE LEVEL OF MORTALITY

PERCENTILE	STANDARDISED MORTALITY RATIO	
	MEN	WOMEN
10th	67.6	70.6
20th	78.4	83.1
30th	86.2	89.7
40th	93.6	94.6
50th	99.7	99.2
60th	105.7	104.5
70th	112.7	109.5
80th	122.3	117.8
90th	139.0	131.5
LOWEST SMR	0.0	0.0
HIGHEST SMR	322.9	351.1
NUMBER OF AREAS WITH ZERO DEATHS	5	3

NUMBER OF LOCAL AUTHORITY AREAS SHOWN ON MAP BY CATEGORY – BASED ON STANDARDISED MORTALITY RATIO (SMR) DURING 1968–78

CATEGORY	NUMBER OF AREAS	
	MEN	WOMEN
SMR SIGNIFICANTLY HIGH, IN TOP TENTH	31	47
SMR SIGNIFICANTLY HIGH, NOT IN TOP TENTH	14	10
SMR NOT SIGNIFICANTLY HIGH, IN TOP TENTH	100	89
SMR NOT SIGNIFICANTLY LOW, IN BOTTOM TENTH	106	110
SMR SIGNIFICANTLY LOW, NOT IN BOTTOM TENTH	15	17
SMR SIGNIFICANTLY LOW, IN BOTTOM TENTH	31	27

ANY AREA WITH A HIGH SMR, BUT WHERE LESS THAN 4 DEATHS OCCURRED IS NOT MAPPED

MORTALITY FROM CANCER OF THE RECTUM
IN ENGLAND AND WALES DURING 1968–78

NUMBER OF DEATHS DURING 1968–78 AND AVERAGE ANNUAL DEATH RATES PER MILLION BY SEX AND AGE GROUPS

AGE GROUP (YEARS)	MEN		WOMEN	
	NUMBER OF DEATHS	RATE PER MILLION	NUMBER OF DEATHS	RATE PER MILLION
0	0	0.0	0	0.0
1–4	0	0.0	0	0.0
5–14	0	0.0	0	0.0
15–24	29	1	9	0.2
25–34	148	4	95	3
35–44	628	20	482	15
45–54	2,668	82	2,049	61
55–64	7,357	242	5,002	149
65–74	12,613	653	8,924	335
75+	11,484	1,418	14,060	808
ALL AGES	34,927	134	30,621	111

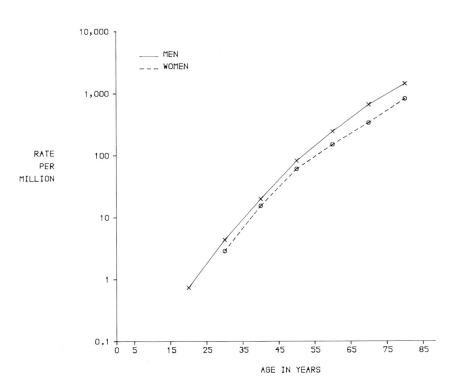

VALUES OF THE STANDARDISED MORTALITY RATIO (SMR) WHICH DIVIDE THE 1366 LOCAL AUTHORITY AREAS INTO TENTHS ACCORDING TO THE LEVEL OF MORTALITY

PERCENTILE	STANDARDISED MORTALITY RATIO	
	MEN	WOMEN
10th	58.6	54.7
20th	72.4	70.1
30th	81.2	80.8
40th	89.1	88.9
50th	97.3	96.3
60th	104.7	103.4
70th	113.8	111.9
80th	124.5	124.0
90th	142.3	139.7
LOWEST SMR	0.0	0.0
HIGHEST SMR	316.0	266.5
NUMBER OF AREAS WITH ZERO DEATHS	21	20

NUMBER OF LOCAL AUTHORITY AREAS SHOWN ON MAP BY CATEGORY – BASED ON STANDARDISED MORTALITY RATIO (SMR) DURING 1968–78

CATEGORY	NUMBER OF AREAS	
	MEN	WOMEN
SMR SIGNIFICANTLY HIGH, IN TOP TENTH	42	17
SMR SIGNIFICANTLY HIGH, NOT IN TOP TENTH	26	13
SMR NOT SIGNIFICANTLY HIGH, IN TOP TENTH	87	109
SMR NOT SIGNIFICANTLY LOW, IN BOTTOM TENTH	109	119
SMR SIGNIFICANTLY LOW, NOT IN BOTTOM TENTH	33	13
SMR SIGNIFICANTLY LOW, IN BOTTOM TENTH	28	18

ANY AREA WITH A HIGH SMR, BUT WHERE LESS THAN 4 DEATHS OCCURRED IS NOT MAPPED

MORTALITY FROM CANCER OF THE PANCREAS
IN ENGLAND AND WALES DURING 1968–78

NUMBER OF DEATHS DURING 1968–78 AND AVERAGE ANNUAL DEATH RATES PER MILLION BY SEX AND AGE GROUPS

AGE GROUP (YEARS)	MEN		WOMEN	
	NUMBER OF DEATHS	RATE PER MILLION	NUMBER OF DEATHS	RATE PER MILLION
0	0	0.0	0	0.0
1–4	1	0.1	0	0.0
5–14	0	0.0	2	0.1
15–24	10	0.3	7	0.2
25–34	119	4	73	2
35–44	618	20	374	12
45–54	2,875	88	1,786	53
55–64	7,808	257	4,914	146
65–74	11,522	597	9,253	347
75+	7,842	968	11,526	663
ALL AGES	30,795	118	27,935	101

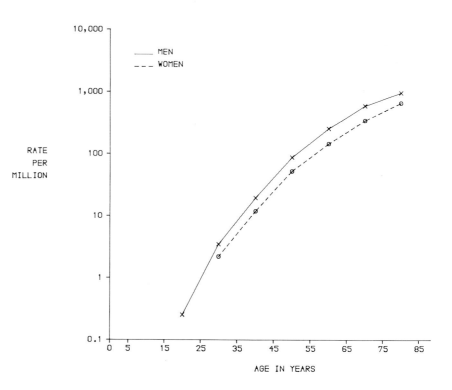

VALUES OF THE STANDARDISED MORTALITY RATIO (SMR) WHICH DIVIDE THE 1366 LOCAL AUTHORITY AREAS INTO TENTHS ACCORDING TO THE LEVEL OF MORTALITY

PERCENTILE	STANDARDISED MORTALITY RATIO	
	MEN	WOMEN
10th	56.1	56.5
20th	71.0	71.7
30th	80.4	83.4
40th	88.6	91.2
50th	96.8	98.8
60th	103.8	104.9
70th	112.2	112.6
80th	122.2	123.2
90th	142.0	142.7
LOWEST SMR	0.0	0.0
HIGHEST SMR	399.3	281.2
NUMBER OF AREAS WITH ZERO DEATHS	24	31

NUMBER OF LOCAL AUTHORITY AREAS SHOWN ON MAP BY CATEGORY – BASED ON STANDARDISED MORTALITY RATIO (SMR) DURING 1968–78

CATEGORY	NUMBER OF AREAS	
	MEN	WOMEN
SMR SIGNIFICANTLY HIGH, IN TOP TENTH	35	20
SMR SIGNIFICANTLY HIGH, NOT IN TOP TENTH	10	5
SMR NOT SIGNIFICANTLY HIGH, IN TOP TENTH	91	101
SMR NOT SIGNIFICANTLY LOW, IN BOTTOM TENTH	116	108
SMR SIGNIFICANTLY LOW, NOT IN BOTTOM TENTH	14	8
SMR SIGNIFICANTLY LOW, IN BOTTOM TENTH	21	29

ANY AREA WITH A HIGH SMR, BUT WHERE LESS THAN 4 DEATHS OCCURRED IS NOT MAPPED

MORTALITY FROM CANCER OF THE LUNG
IN ENGLAND AND WALES DURING 1968–78

NUMBER OF DEATHS DURING 1968–78 AND AVERAGE ANNUAL DEATH RATES PER MILLION BY SEX AND AGE GROUPS

AGE GROUP (YEARS)	MEN		WOMEN	
	NUMBER OF DEATHS	RATE PER MILLION	NUMBER OF DEATHS	RATE PER MILLION
0	1	0.2	0	0.0
1–4	6	0.3	3	0.2
5–14	5	0.1	4	0.1
15–24	80	2	30	1
25–34	540	16	208	6
35–44	3,758	119	1,524	49
45–54	25,369	778	8,307	246
55–64	81,788	2,690	18,860	562
65–74	116,803	6,049	23,335	876
75+	54,689	6,750	15,961	918
ALL AGES	283,039	1,086	68,232	247

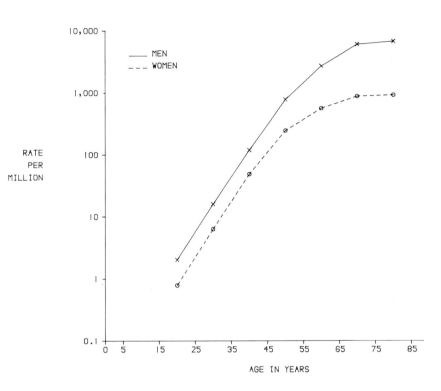

VALUES OF THE STANDARDISED MORTALITY RATIO (SMR) WHICH DIVIDE THE 1366 LOCAL AUTHORITY AREAS INTO TENTHS ACCORDING TO THE LEVEL OF MORTALITY

PERCENTILE	STANDARDISED MORTALITY RATIO	
	MEN	WOMEN
10th	64.1	52.3
20th	71.7	64.2
30th	78.2	72.5
40th	82.9	79.5
50th	87.1	87.2
60th	91.6	93.9
70th	96.5	101.4
80th	102.2	111.0
90th	112.5	124.1
LOWEST SMR	18.1	0.0
HIGHEST SMR	200.0	267.0
NUMBER OF AREAS WITH ZERO DEATHS	0	9

NUMBER OF LOCAL AUTHORITY AREAS SHOWN ON MAP BY CATEGORY – BASED ON STANDARDISED MORTALITY RATIO (SMR) DURING 1968–78

CATEGORY	NUMBER OF AREAS	
	MEN	WOMEN
SMR SIGNIFICANTLY HIGH, IN TOP TENTH	95	58
SMR SIGNIFICANTLY HIGH, NOT IN TOP TENTH	12	18
SMR NOT SIGNIFICANTLY HIGH, IN TOP TENTH	42	75
SMR NOT SIGNIFICANTLY LOW, IN BOTTOM TENTH	14	58
SMR SIGNIFICANTLY LOW, NOT IN BOTTOM TENTH	343	109
SMR SIGNIFICANTLY LOW, IN BOTTOM TENTH	123	79

ANY AREA WITH A HIGH SMR, BUT WHERE LESS THAN 4 DEATHS OCCURRED IS NOT MAPPED

MORTALITY FROM CANCER OF THE BREAST
IN ENGLAND AND WALES DURING 1968–78

NUMBER OF DEATHS DURING 1968–78 AND AVERAGE ANNUAL DEATH RATES PER MILLION BY SEX AND AGE GROUPS

AGE GROUP (YEARS)	MEN		WOMEN	
	NUMBER OF DEATHS	RATE PER MILLION	NUMBER OF DEATHS	RATE PER MILLION
0	0	0.0	0	0.0
1–4	0	0.0	0	0.0
5–14	0	0.0	2	0.1
15–24	0	0.0	56	1
25–34	6	0.2	1,338	41
35–44	19	1	7,427	237
45–54	76	2	21,215	628
55–64	216	7	30,853	919
65–74	297	15	31,814	1,194
75+	260	32	30,931	1,778
ALL AGES	874	3	123,636	448

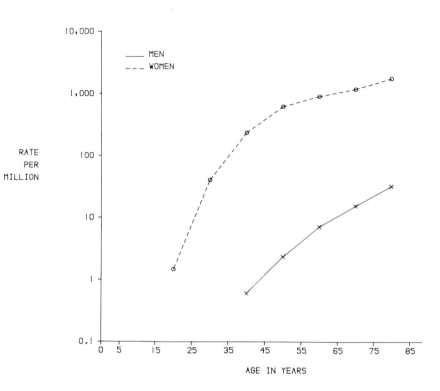

VALUES OF THE STANDARDISED MORTALITY RATIO (SMR) WHICH DIVIDE THE 1366 LOCAL AUTHORITY AREAS INTO TENTHS ACCORDING TO THE LEVEL OF MORTALITY

PERCENTILE	STANDARDISED MORTALITY RATIO	
	MEN	WOMEN
10th	—	75.9
20th	—	84.5
30th	—	89.7
40th	—	94.7
50th	—	99.1
60th	—	102.9
70th	—	107.1
80th	—	112.5
90th	—	123.4
LOWEST SMR	—	0.0
HIGHEST SMR	—	324.1
NUMBER OF AREAS WITH ZERO DEATHS	—	4

NUMBER OF LOCAL AUTHORITY AREAS SHOWN ON MAP BY CATEGORY – BASED ON STANDARDISED MORTALITY RATIO (SMR) DURING 1968–78

CATEGORY	NUMBER OF AREAS	
	MEN	WOMEN
SMR SIGNIFICANTLY HIGH, IN TOP TENTH	—	41
SMR SIGNIFICANTLY HIGH, NOT IN TOP TENTH	—	23
SMR NOT SIGNIFICANTLY HIGH, IN TOP TENTH	—	96
SMR NOT SIGNIFICANTLY LOW, IN BOTTOM TENTH	—	90
SMR SIGNIFICANTLY LOW, NOT IN BOTTOM TENTH	—	22
SMR SIGNIFICANTLY LOW, IN BOTTOM TENTH	—	47

ANY AREA WITH A HIGH SMR, BUT WHERE LESS THAN 4 DEATHS OCCURRED IS NOT MAPPED

MORTALITY FROM CANCER OF THE CERVIX
IN ENGLAND AND WALES DURING 1968–78

NUMBER OF DEATHS DURING 1968–78 AND AVERAGE ANNUAL DEATH RATES PER MILLION BY SEX AND AGE GROUPS

AGE GROUP (YEARS)	MEN		WOMEN	
	NUMBER OF DEATHS	RATE PER MILLION	NUMBER OF DEATHS	RATE PER MILLION
0	—	—	0	0.0
1–4	—	—	0	0.0
5–14	—	—	0	0.0
15–24	—	—	53	1
25–34	—	—	566	17
35–44	—	—	1,801	58
45–54	—	—	5,426	161
55–64	—	—	6,585	196
65–74	—	—	5,615	211
75+	—	—	4,645	267
ALL AGES	—	—	24,691	90

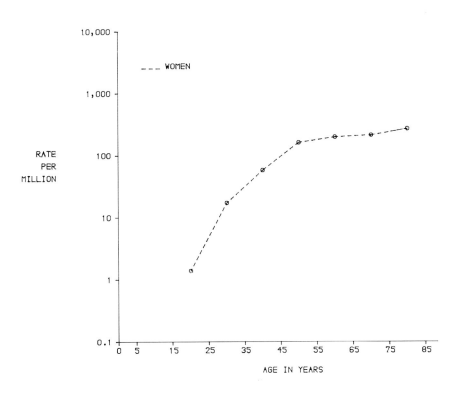

VALUES OF THE STANDARDISED MORTALITY RATIO (SMR) WHICH DIVIDE THE 1366 LOCAL AUTHORITY AREAS INTO TENTHS ACCORDING TO THE LEVEL OF MORTALITY

PERCENTILE	STANDARDISED MORTALITY RATIO	
	MEN	WOMEN
10th	—	45.3
20th	—	64.7
30th	—	75.5
40th	—	84.6
50th	—	93.9
60th	—	103.3
70th	—	116.6
80th	—	131.9
90th	—	157.2
LOWEST SMR	—	0.0
HIGHEST SMR	—	468.5
NUMBER OF AREAS WITH ZERO DEATHS	—	48

NUMBER OF LOCAL AUTHORITY AREAS SHOWN ON MAP BY CATEGORY – BASED ON STANDARDISED MORTALITY RATIO (SMR) DURING 1968–78

CATEGORY	NUMBER OF AREAS	
	MEN	WOMEN
SMR SIGNIFICANTLY HIGH, IN TOP TENTH	—	44
SMR SIGNIFICANTLY HIGH, NOT IN TOP TENTH	—	31
SMR NOT SIGNIFICANTLY HIGH, IN TOP TENTH	—	77
SMR NOT SIGNIFICANTLY LOW, IN BOTTOM TENTH	—	107
SMR SIGNIFICANTLY LOW, NOT IN BOTTOM TENTH	—	44
SMR SIGNIFICANTLY LOW, IN BOTTOM TENTH	—	30

ANY AREA WITH A HIGH SMR, BUT WHERE LESS THAN 4 DEATHS OCCURRED IS NOT MAPPED

MORTALITY FROM OTHER CANCER OF THE UTERUS
IN ENGLAND AND WALES DURING 1968–78

NUMBER OF DEATHS DURING 1968–78 AND AVERAGE ANNUAL DEATH RATES PER MILLION BY SEX AND AGE GROUPS

AGE GROUP (YEARS)	MEN		WOMEN	
	NUMBER OF DEATHS	RATE PER MILLION	NUMBER OF DEATHS	RATE PER MILLION
0	—	—	0	0.0
1–4	—	—	3	0.2
5–14	—	—	3	0.1
15–24	—	—	7	0.2
25–34	—	—	38	1
35–44	—	—	213	7
45–54	—	—	1,472	44
55–64	—	—	4,024	120
65–74	—	—	5,683	213
75+	—	—	5,357	308
ALL AGES	—	—	16,800	61

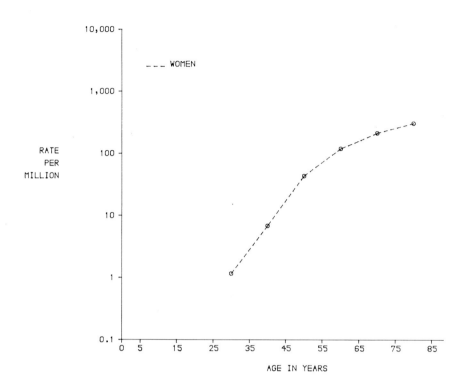

VALUES OF THE STANDARDISED MORTALITY RATIO (SMR) WHICH DIVIDE THE 1366 LOCAL AUTHORITY AREAS INTO TENTHS ACCORDING TO THE LEVEL OF MORTALITY

PERCENTILE	STANDARDISED MORTALITY RATIO	
	MEN	WOMEN
10th	—	45.0
20th	—	65.3
30th	—	78.1
40th	—	88.8
50th	—	98.2
60th	—	108.3
70th	—	120.6
80th	—	137.4
90th	—	168.5
LOWEST SMR	—	0.0
HIGHEST SMR	—	700.6
NUMBER OF AREAS WITH ZERO DEATHS	—	67

NUMBER OF LOCAL AUTHORITY AREAS SHOWN ON MAP BY CATEGORY – BASED ON STANDARDISED MORTALITY RATIO (SMR) DURING 1968–78

CATEGORY	NUMBER OF AREAS	
	MEN	WOMEN
SMR SIGNIFICANTLY HIGH, IN TOP TENTH	—	40
SMR SIGNIFICANTLY HIGH, NOT IN TOP TENTH	—	9
SMR NOT SIGNIFICANTLY HIGH, IN TOP TENTH	—	66
SMR NOT SIGNIFICANTLY LOW, IN BOTTOM TENTH	—	119
SMR SIGNIFICANTLY LOW, NOT IN BOTTOM TENTH	—	9
SMR SIGNIFICANTLY LOW, IN BOTTOM TENTH	—	18

ANY AREA WITH A HIGH SMR, BUT WHERE LESS THAN 4 DEATHS OCCURRED IS NOT MAPPED

MORTALITY FROM CANCER OF THE OVARY
IN ENGLAND AND WALES DURING 1968–78

NUMBER OF DEATHS DURING 1968–78 AND AVERAGE ANNUAL DEATH RATES PER MILLION BY SEX AND AGE GROUPS

AGE GROUP (YEARS)	MEN		WOMEN	
	NUMBER OF DEATHS	RATE PER MILLION	NUMBER OF DEATHS	RATE PER MILLION
0	—	—	0	0.0
1–4	—	—	3	0.2
5–14	—	—	35	1
15–24	—	—	173	5
25–34	—	—	386	12
35–44	—	—	1,881	60
45–54	—	—	7,039	209
55–64	—	—	11,046	329
65–74	—	—	11,606	436
75+	—	—	7,514	432
ALL AGES	—	—	39,683	144

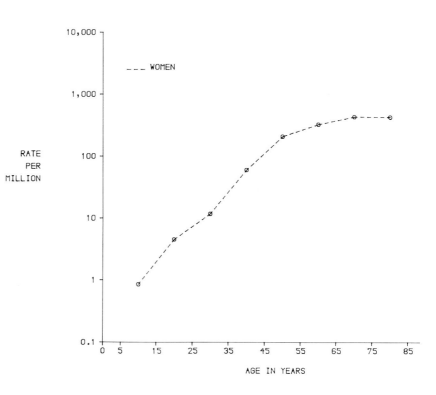

VALUES OF THE STANDARDISED MORTALITY RATIO (SMR) WHICH DIVIDE THE 1366 LOCAL AUTHORITY AREAS INTO TENTHS ACCORDING TO THE LEVEL OF MORTALITY

PERCENTILE	STANDARDISED MORTALITY RATIO	
	MEN	WOMEN
10th	—	61.8
20th	—	75.2
30th	—	85.7
40th	—	92.1
50th	—	98.8
60th	—	105.6
70th	—	114.7
80th	—	125.4
90th	—	144.1
LOWEST SMR	—	0.0
HIGHEST SMR	—	480.0
NUMBER OF AREAS WITH ZERO DEATHS	—	20

NUMBER OF LOCAL AUTHORITY AREAS SHOWN ON MAP BY CATEGORY – BASED ON STANDARDISED MORTALITY RATIO (SMR) DURING 1968–78

CATEGORY	NUMBER OF AREAS	
	MEN	WOMEN
SMR SIGNIFICANTLY HIGH, IN TOP TENTH	—	45
SMR SIGNIFICANTLY HIGH, NOT IN TOP TENTH	—	14
SMR NOT SIGNIFICANTLY HIGH, IN TOP TENTH	—	88
SMR NOT SIGNIFICANTLY LOW, IN BOTTOM TENTH	—	115
SMR SIGNIFICANTLY LOW, NOT IN BOTTOM TENTH	—	19
SMR SIGNIFICANTLY LOW, IN BOTTOM TENTH	—	22

ANY AREA WITH A HIGH SMR, BUT WHERE LESS THAN 4 DEATHS OCCURRED IS NOT MAPPED

MORTALITY FROM CANCER OF THE BLADDER
IN ENGLAND AND WALES DURING 1968–78

NUMBER OF DEATHS DURING 1968–78 AND AVERAGE ANNUAL
DEATH RATES PER MILLION BY SEX AND AGE GROUPS

AGE GROUP (YEARS)	MEN		WOMEN	
	NUMBER OF DEATHS	RATE PER MILLION	NUMBER OF DEATHS	RATE PER MILLION
0	2	0.5	0	0.0
1–4	11	1	3	0.2
5–14	7	0.2	4	0.1
15–24	3	0.1	1	0.0
25–34	20	1	16	0.5
35–44	239	8	118	4
45–54	1,611	49	568	17
55–64	5,947	196	1,844	55
65–74	11,930	618	3,950	148
75+	11,057	1,365	6,663	383
ALL AGES	30,827	118	13,167	48

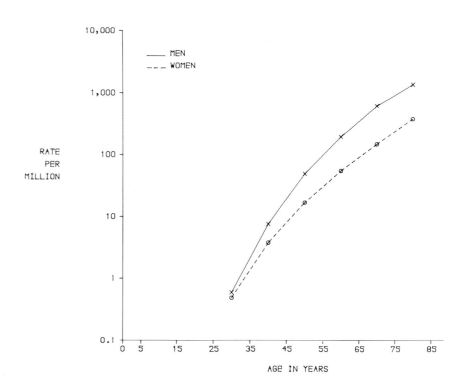

VALUES OF THE STANDARDISED MORTALITY RATIO
(SMR) WHICH DIVIDE THE 1366 LOCAL AUTHORITY
AREAS INTO TENTHS ACCORDING TO THE LEVEL
OF MORTALITY

PERCENTILE	STANDARDISED MORTALITY RATIO	
	MEN	WOMEN
10th	49.6	22.9
20th	64.8	52.3
30th	75.0	68.6
40th	84.8	81.3
50th	93.2	92.3
60th	100.1	103.4
70th	107.9	116.9
80th	117.5	132.6
90th	134.6	160.8
LOWEST SMR	0.0	0.0
HIGHEST SMR	300.4	633.0
NUMBER OF AREAS WITH ZERO DEATHS	31	128

NUMBER OF LOCAL AUTHORITY AREAS SHOWN ON MAP BY CATEGORY –
BASED ON STANDARDISED MORTALITY RATIO (SMR) DURING 1968–78

CATEGORY	NUMBER OF AREAS	
	MEN	WOMEN
SMR SIGNIFICANTLY HIGH, IN TOP TENTH	22	28
SMR SIGNIFICANTLY HIGH, NOT IN TOP TENTH	21	9
SMR NOT SIGNIFICANTLY HIGH, IN TOP TENTH	102	67
SMR NOT SIGNIFICANTLY LOW, IN BOTTOM TENTH	94	129
SMR SIGNIFICANTLY LOW, NOT IN BOTTOM TENTH	10	11
SMR SIGNIFICANTLY LOW, IN BOTTOM TENTH	43	8

ANY AREA WITH A HIGH SMR, BUT WHERE LESS THAN 4 DEATHS OCCURRED IS
NOT MAPPED

46

MORTALITY FROM CANCER OF THE PROSTATE
IN ENGLAND AND WALES DURING 1968-78

NUMBER OF DEATHS DURING 1968-78 AND AVERAGE ANNUAL
DEATH RATES PER MILLION BY SEX AND AGE GROUPS

AGE GROUP (YEARS)	MEN		WOMEN	
	NUMBER OF DEATHS	RATE PER MILLION	NUMBER OF DEATHS	RATE PER MILLION
0	0	0.0	—	—
1-4	6	0.3	—	—
5-14	2	0.1	—	—
15-24	8	0.2	—	—
25-34	3	0.1	—	—
35-44	36	1	—	—
45-54	597	18	—	—
55-64	4,777	157	—	—
65-74	16,434	851	—	—
75+	25,105	3,099	—	—
ALL AGES	46,968	180	—	—

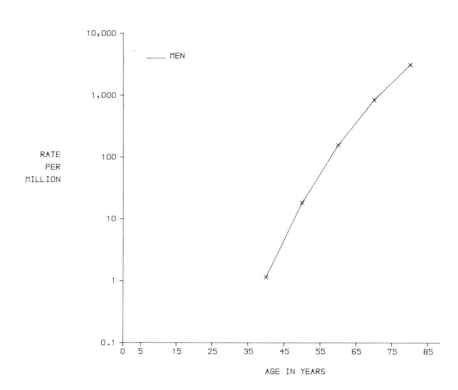

VALUES OF THE STANDARDISED MORTALITY RATIO
(SMR) WHICH DIVIDE THE 1366 LOCAL AUTHORITY
AREAS INTO TENTHS ACCORDING TO THE LEVEL
OF MORTALITY

PERCENTILE	STANDARDISED MORTALITY RATIO	
	MEN	WOMEN
10th	63.3	—
20th	77.9	—
30th	86.5	—
40th	93.6	—
50th	99.7	—
60th	105.4	—
70th	112.2	—
80th	121.5	—
90th	136.4	—
LOWEST SMR	0.0	—
HIGHEST SMR	238.7	—
NUMBER OF AREAS WITH ZERO DEATHS	6	—

NUMBER OF LOCAL AUTHORITY AREAS SHOWN ON MAP BY CATEGORY –
BASED ON STANDARDISED MORTALITY RATIO (SMR) DURING 1968-78

CATEGORY	NUMBER OF AREAS	
	MEN	WOMEN
SMR SIGNIFICANTLY HIGH, IN TOP TENTH	36	—
SMR SIGNIFICANTLY HIGH, NOT IN TOP TENTH	11	—
SMR NOT SIGNIFICANTLY HIGH, IN TOP TENTH	97	—
SMR NOT SIGNIFICANTLY LOW, IN BOTTOM TENTH	97	—
SMR SIGNIFICANTLY LOW, NOT IN BOTTOM TENTH	20	—
SMR SIGNIFICANTLY LOW, IN BOTTOM TENTH	40	—

ANY AREA WITH A HIGH SMR, BUT WHERE LESS THAN 4 DEATHS OCCURRED IS
NOT MAPPED

MORTALITY FROM MESOTHELIOMA OF THE PLEURA
IN ENGLAND AND WALES DURING 1968-78

NUMBER OF DEATHS DURING 1968-78 AND AVERAGE ANNUAL DEATH RATES PER MILLION BY SEX AND AGE GROUPS

AGE GROUP (YEARS)	MEN		WOMEN	
	NUMBER OF DEATHS	RATE PER MILLION	NUMBER OF DEATHS	RATE PER MILLION
0	0	0.0	0	0.0
1-4	0	0.0	0	0.0
5-14	2	0.0	0	0.0
15-24	3	0.1	8	0.2
25-34	15	0.4	8	0.2
35-44	62	2	25	1
45-54	242	7	64	2
55-64	491	16	138	4
65-74	423	22	144	5
75+	168	21	67	4
ALL AGES	1,406	5	454	2

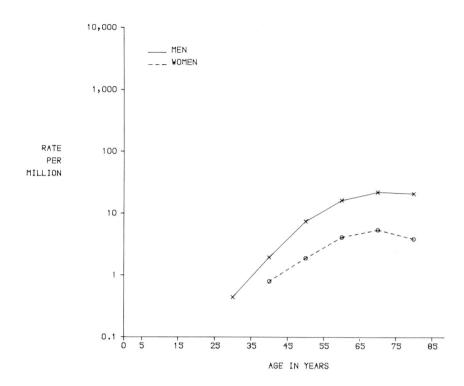

VALUES OF THE STANDARDISED MORTALITY RATIO (SMR) WHICH DIVIDE THE 1366 LOCAL AUTHORITY AREAS INTO TENTHS ACCORDING TO THE LEVEL OF MORTALITY

PERCENTILE	STANDARDISED MORTALITY RATIO	
	MEN	WOMEN
10th	0.0	0.0
20th	0.0	0.0
30th	0.0	0.0
40th	0.0	0.0
50th	0.0	0.0
60th	0.0	0.0
70th	51.9	0.0
80th	117.8	0.0
90th	225.8	251.5
LOWEST SMR	0.0	0.0
HIGHEST SMR	1827.4	2416.2
NUMBER OF AREAS WITH ZERO DEATHS	916	1133

NUMBER OF LOCAL AUTHORITY AREAS SHOWN ON MAP BY CATEGORY – BASED ON STANDARDISED MORTALITY RATIO (SMR) DURING 1968-78

CATEGORY	NUMBER OF AREAS	
	MEN	WOMEN
SMR SIGNIFICANTLY HIGH, IN TOP TENTH	36	15
SMR SIGNIFICANTLY HIGH, NOT IN TOP TENTH	2	1
SMR NOT SIGNIFICANTLY HIGH, IN TOP TENTH	12	2

ANY AREA WITH A HIGH SMR, BUT WHERE LESS THAN 4 DEATHS OCCURRED IS NOT MAPPED

Section 2

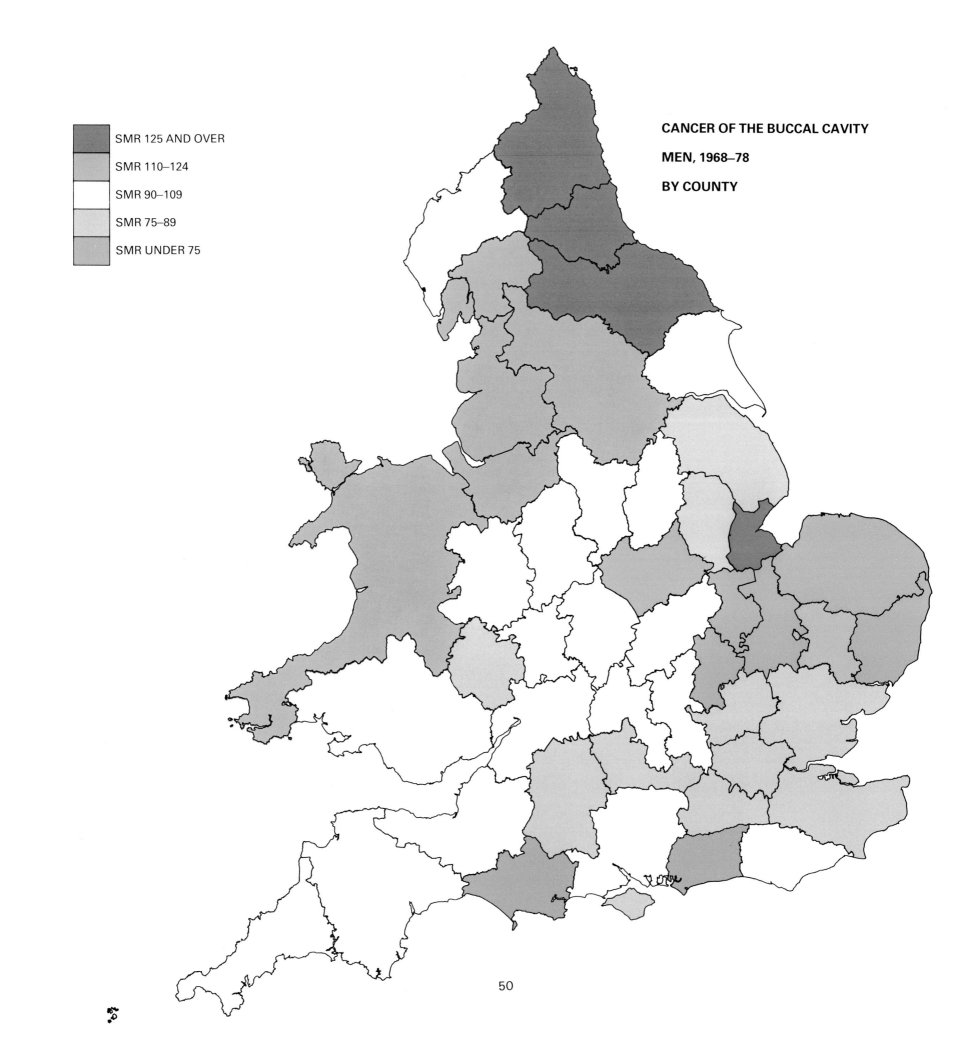

SMR 125 AND OVER

SMR 110–124

SMR 90–109

SMR 75–89

SMR UNDER 75

CANCER OF THE BUCCAL CAVITY

MEN, 1968–78

BY COUNTY

50

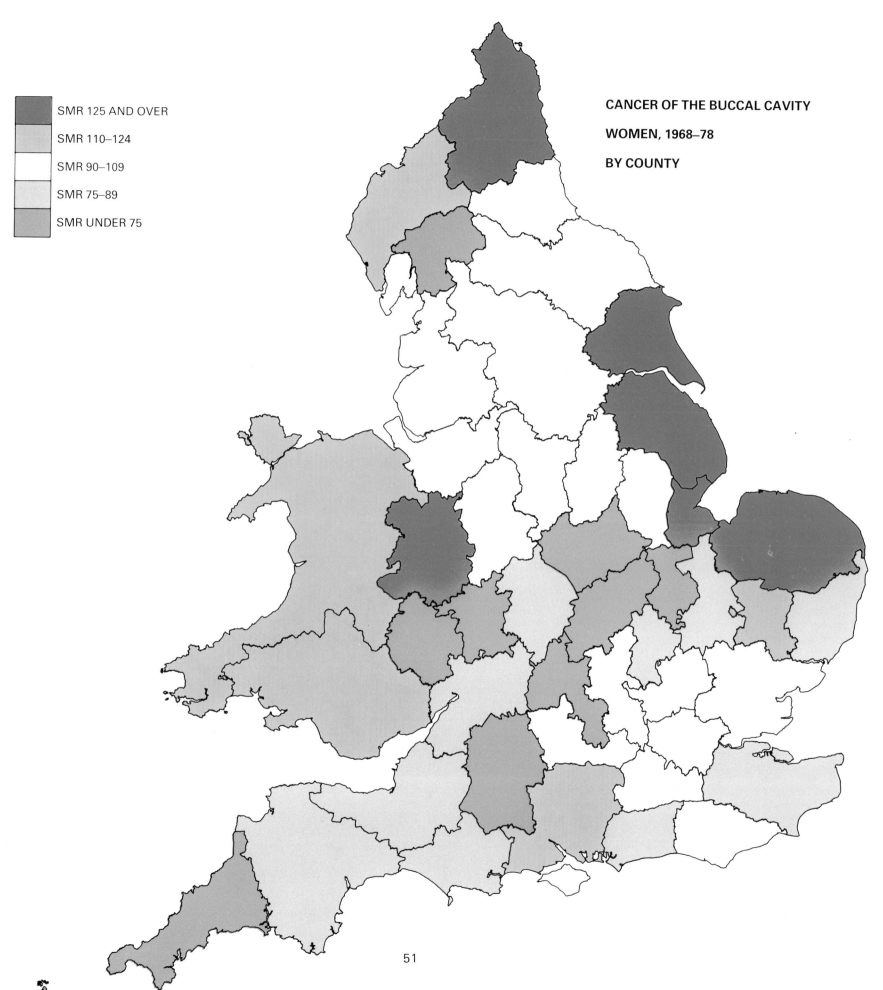

SMR 125 AND OVER

SMR 110–124

SMR 90–109

SMR 75–89

SMR UNDER 75

CANCER OF THE BUCCAL CAVITY

WOMEN, 1968–78

BY COUNTY

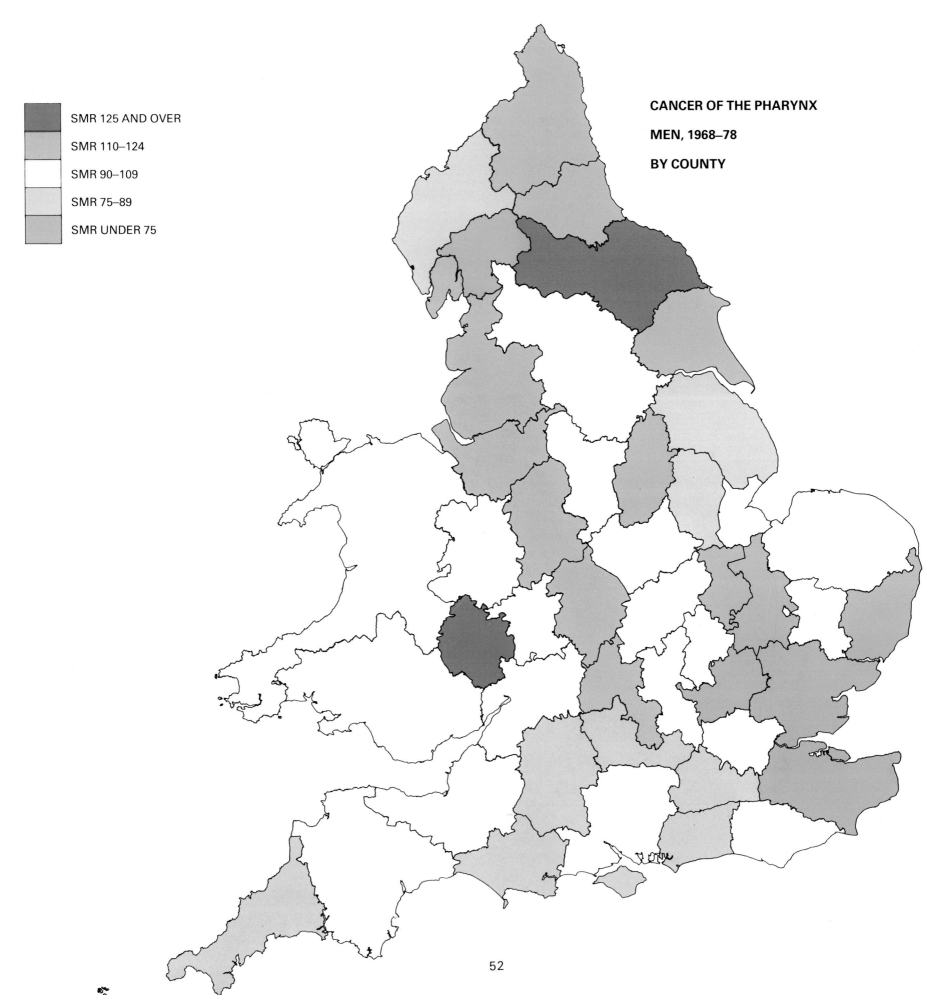

CANCER OF THE PHARYNX

MEN, 1968–78

BY COUNTY

SMR 125 AND OVER

SMR 110–124

SMR 90–109

SMR 75–89

SMR UNDER 75

52

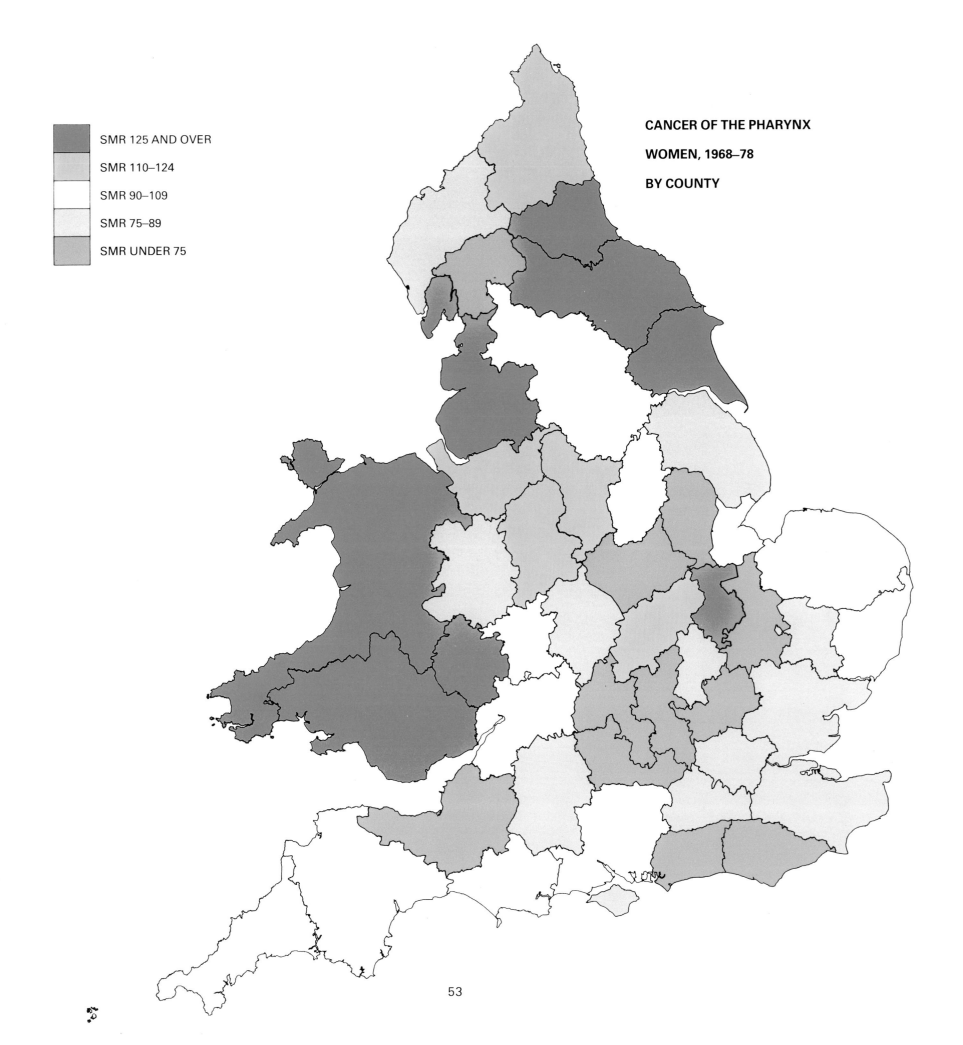

CANCER OF THE PHARYNX

WOMEN, 1968–78

BY COUNTY

SMR 125 AND OVER

SMR 110–124

SMR 90–109

SMR 75–89

SMR UNDER 75

53

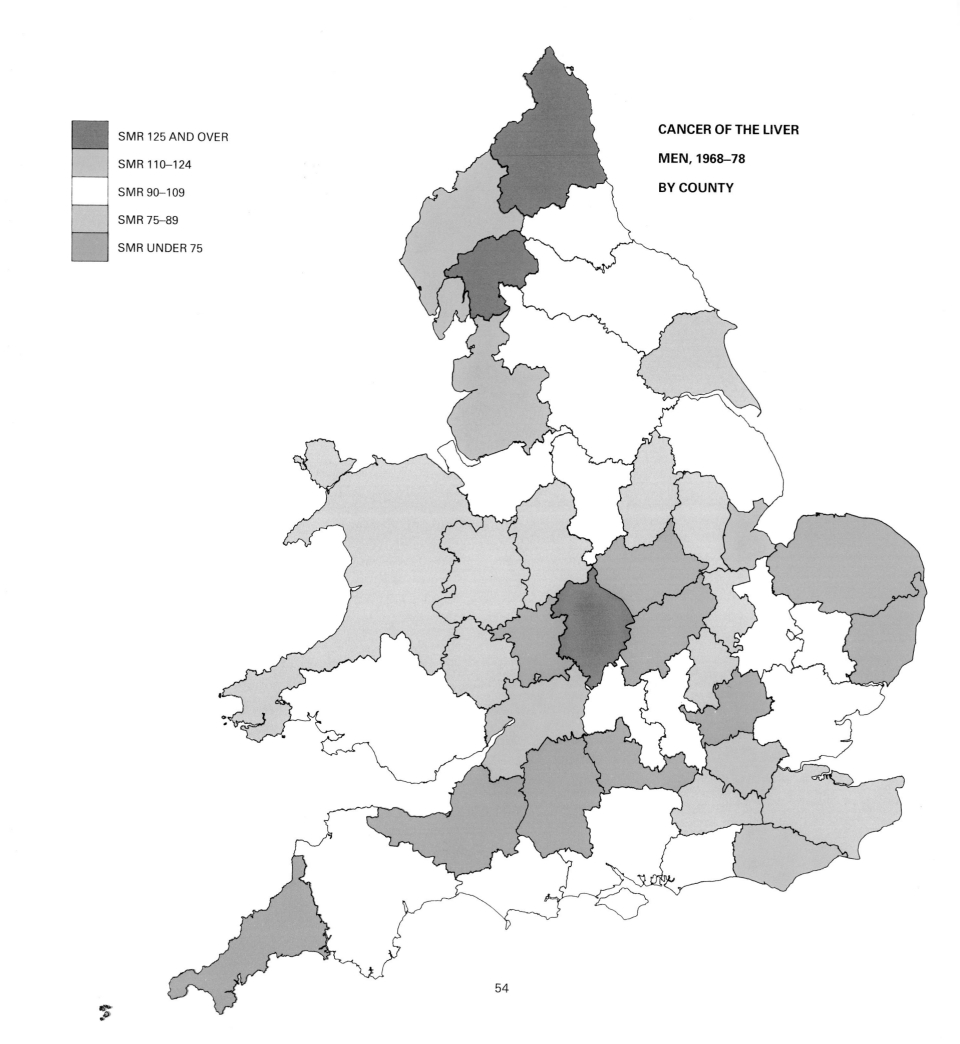

SMR 125 AND OVER

SMR 110–124

SMR 90–109

SMR 75–89

SMR UNDER 75

CANCER OF THE LIVER

MEN, 1968–78

BY COUNTY

54

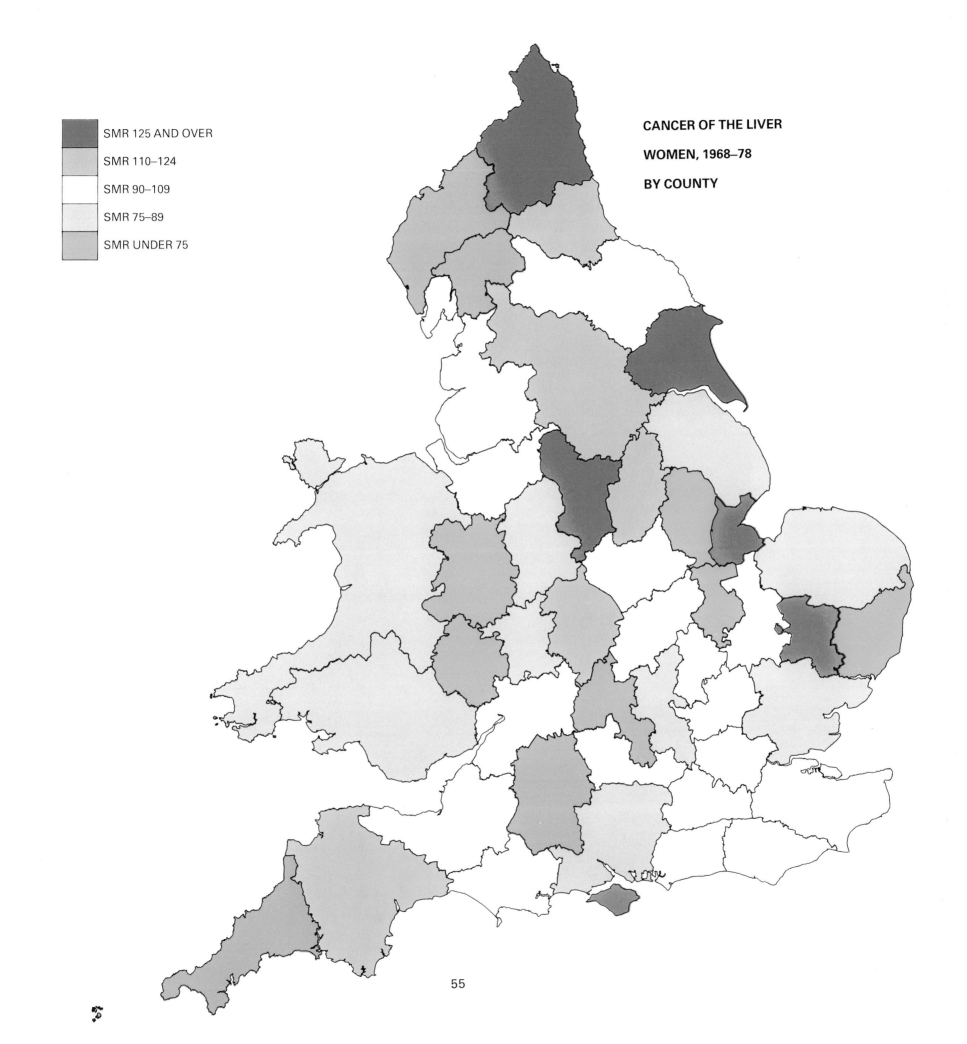

CANCER OF THE LIVER

WOMEN, 1968–78

BY COUNTY

SMR 125 AND OVER

SMR 110–124

SMR 90–109

SMR 75–89

SMR UNDER 75

55

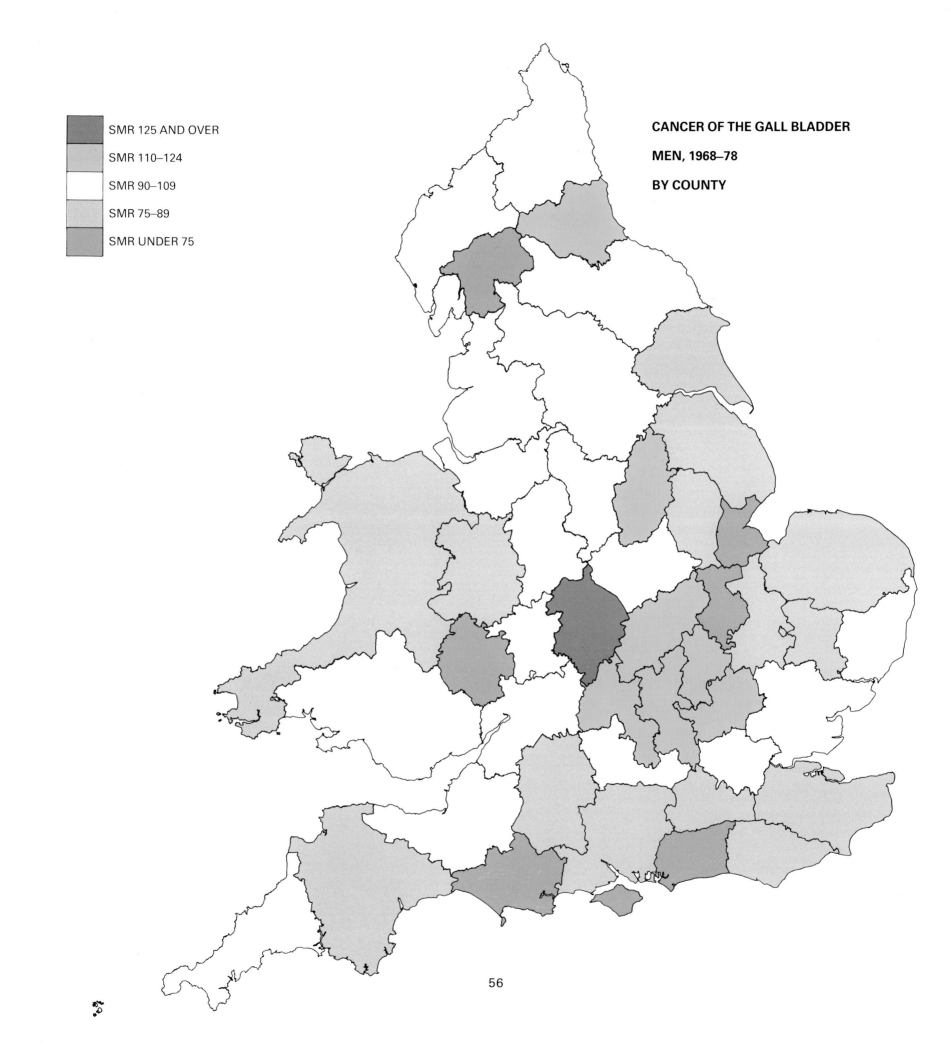

CANCER OF THE GALL BLADDER

MEN, 1968–78

BY COUNTY

SMR 125 AND OVER

SMR 110–124

SMR 90–109

SMR 75–89

SMR UNDER 75

56

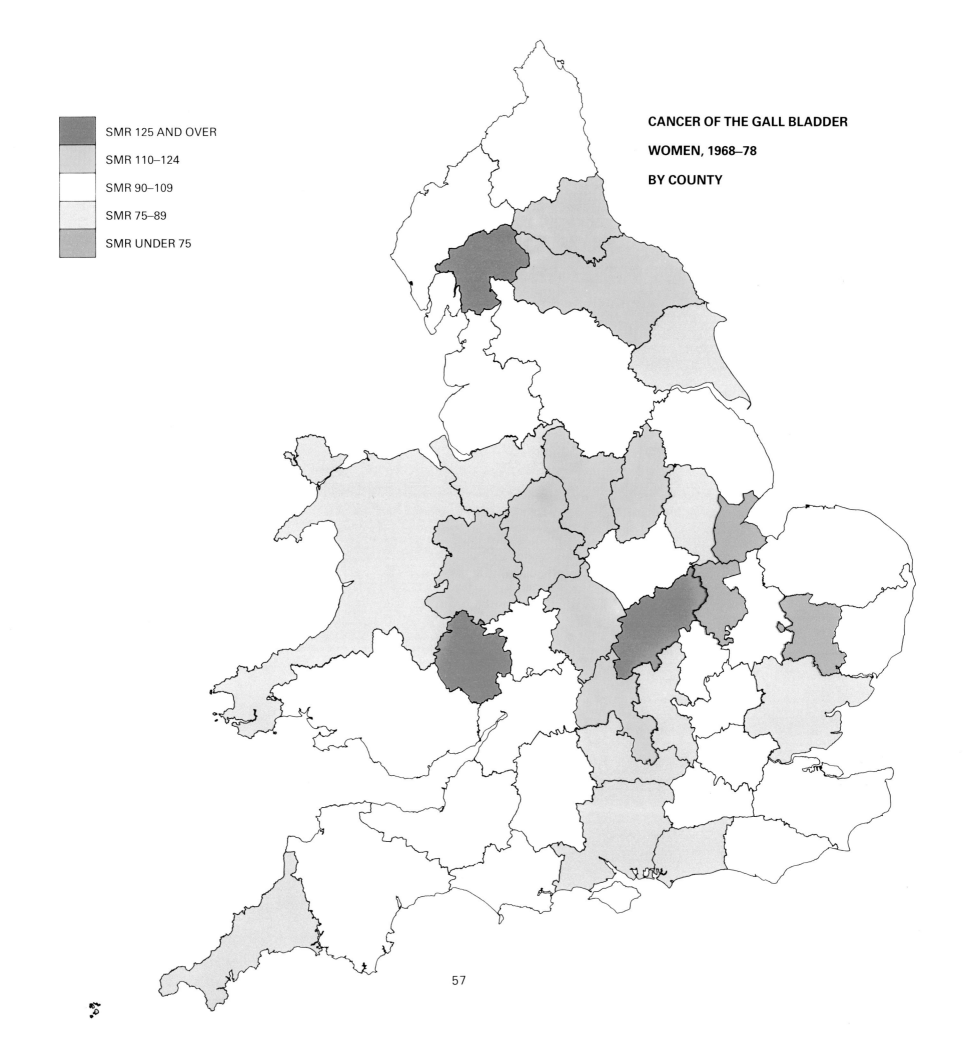

CANCER OF THE GALL BLADDER

WOMEN, 1968–78

BY COUNTY

SMR 125 AND OVER

SMR 110–124

SMR 90–109

SMR 75–89

SMR UNDER 75

57

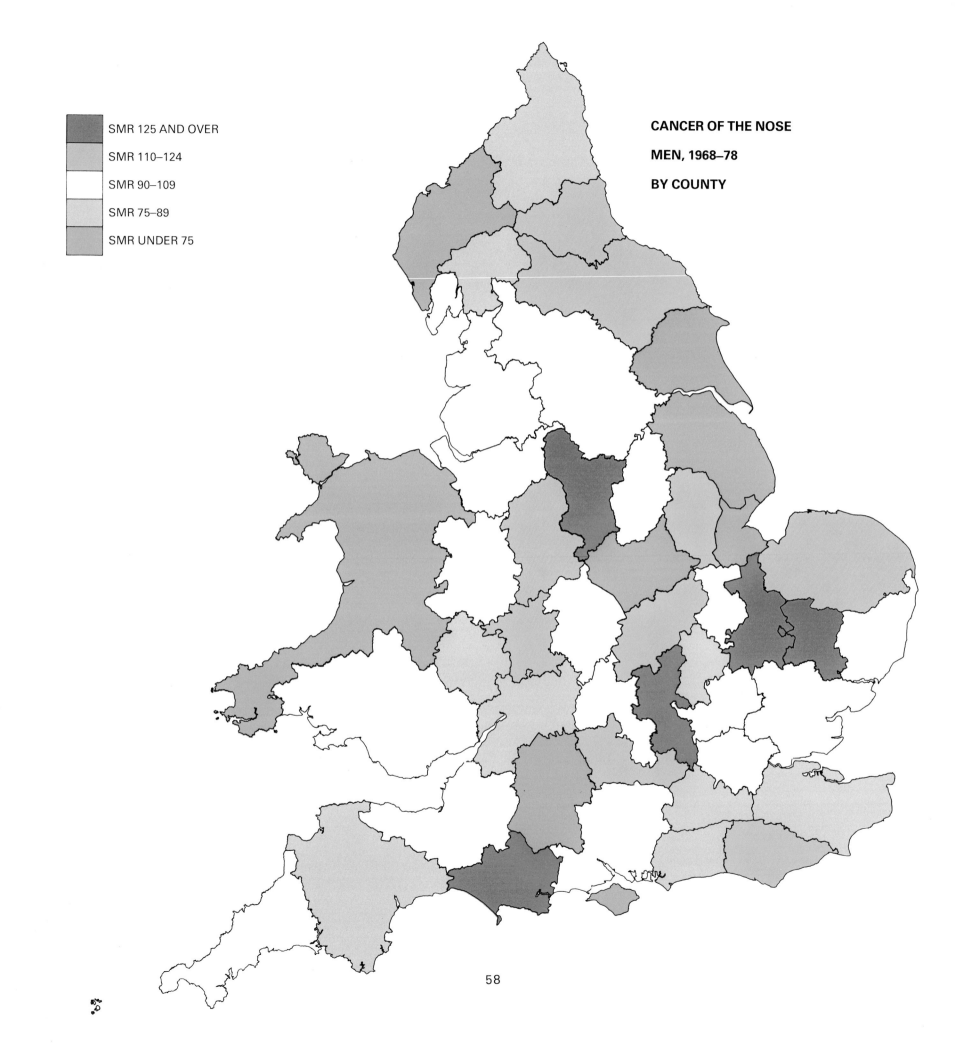

CANCER OF THE NOSE

MEN, 1968–78

BY COUNTY

SMR 125 AND OVER

SMR 110–124

SMR 90–109

SMR 75–89

SMR UNDER 75

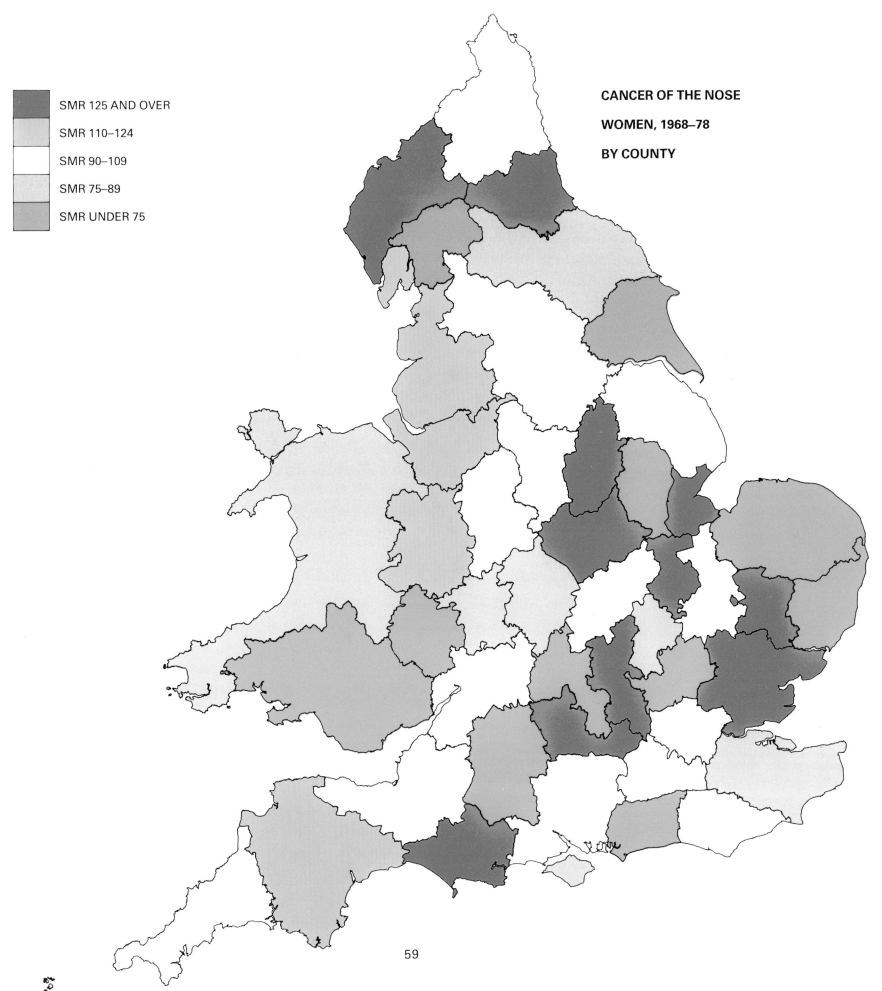

CANCER OF THE NOSE

WOMEN, 1968–78

BY COUNTY

SMR 125 AND OVER

SMR 110–124

SMR 90–109

SMR 75–89

SMR UNDER 75

59

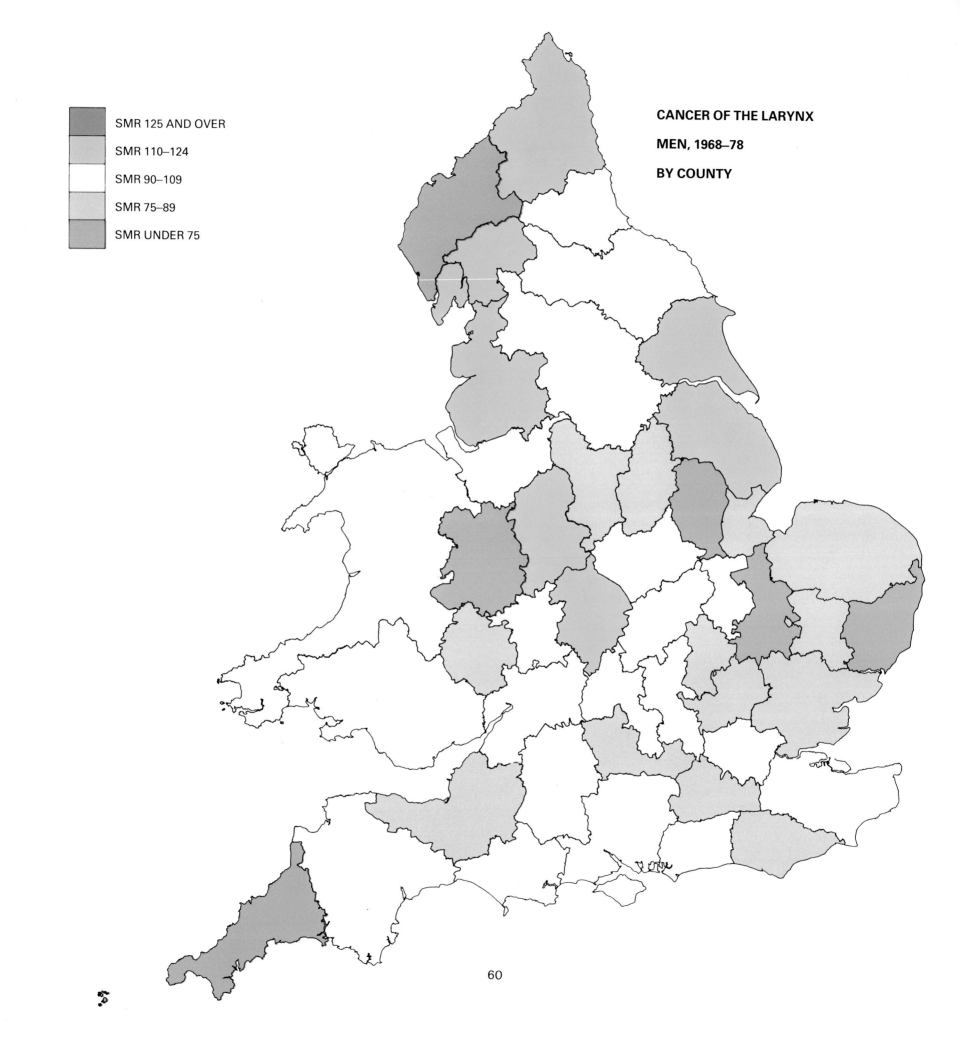

CANCER OF THE LARYNX

MEN, 1968–78

BY COUNTY

SMR 125 AND OVER

SMR 110–124

SMR 90–109

SMR 75–89

SMR UNDER 75

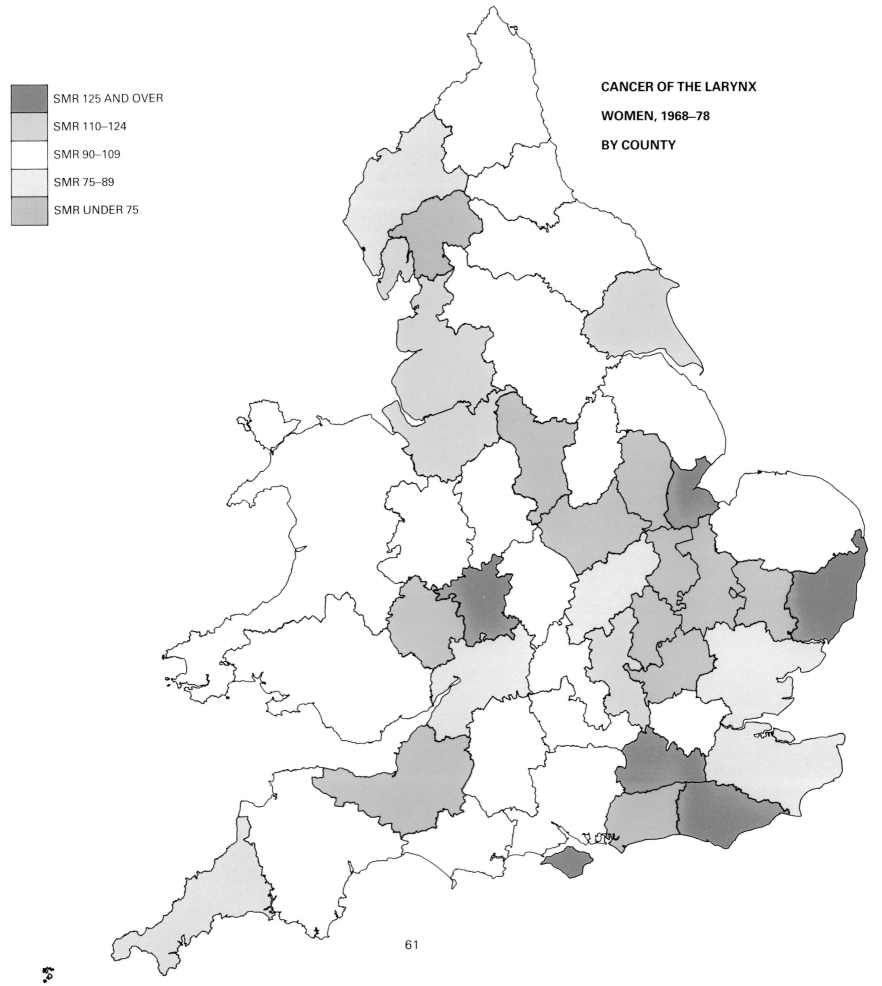

CANCER OF THE LARYNX

WOMEN, 1968–78

BY COUNTY

SMR 125 AND OVER

SMR 110–124

SMR 90–109

SMR 75–89

SMR UNDER 75

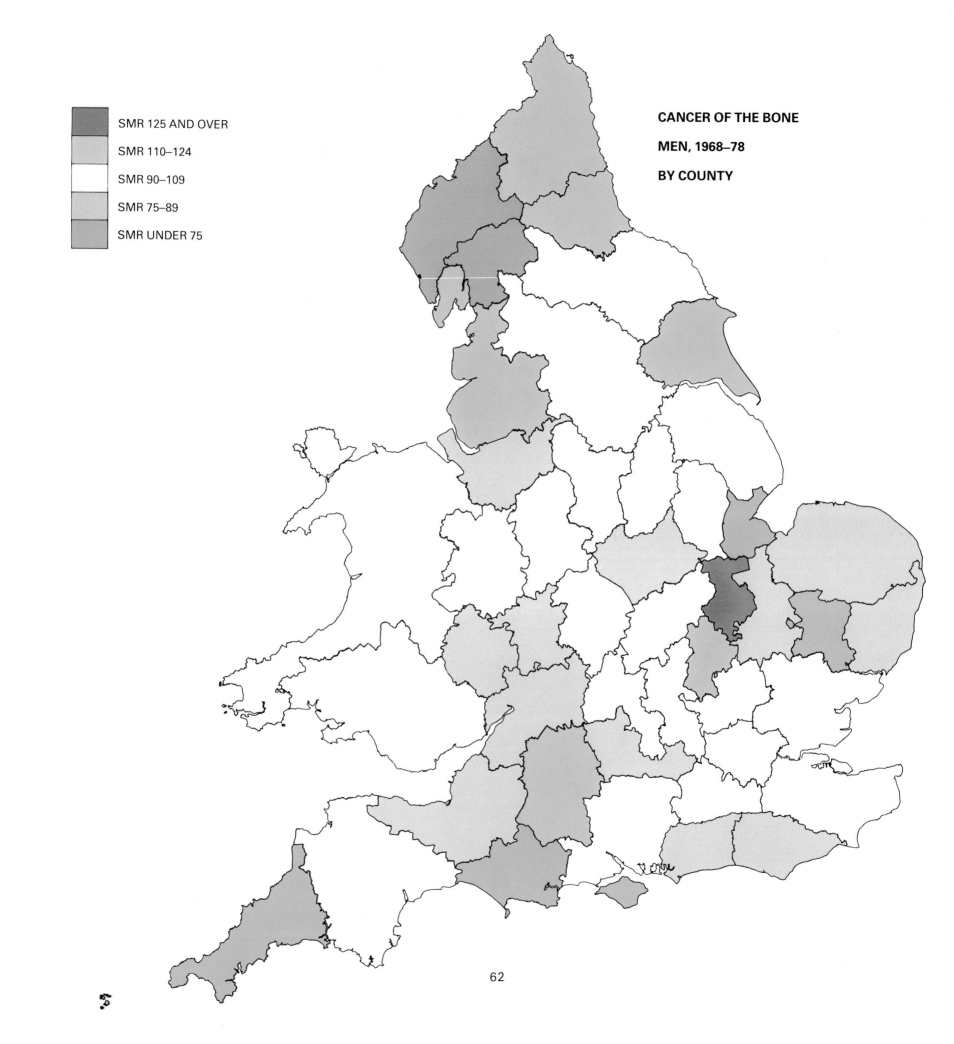

CANCER OF THE BONE

MEN, 1968–78

BY COUNTY

SMR 125 AND OVER

SMR 110–124

SMR 90–109

SMR 75–89

SMR UNDER 75

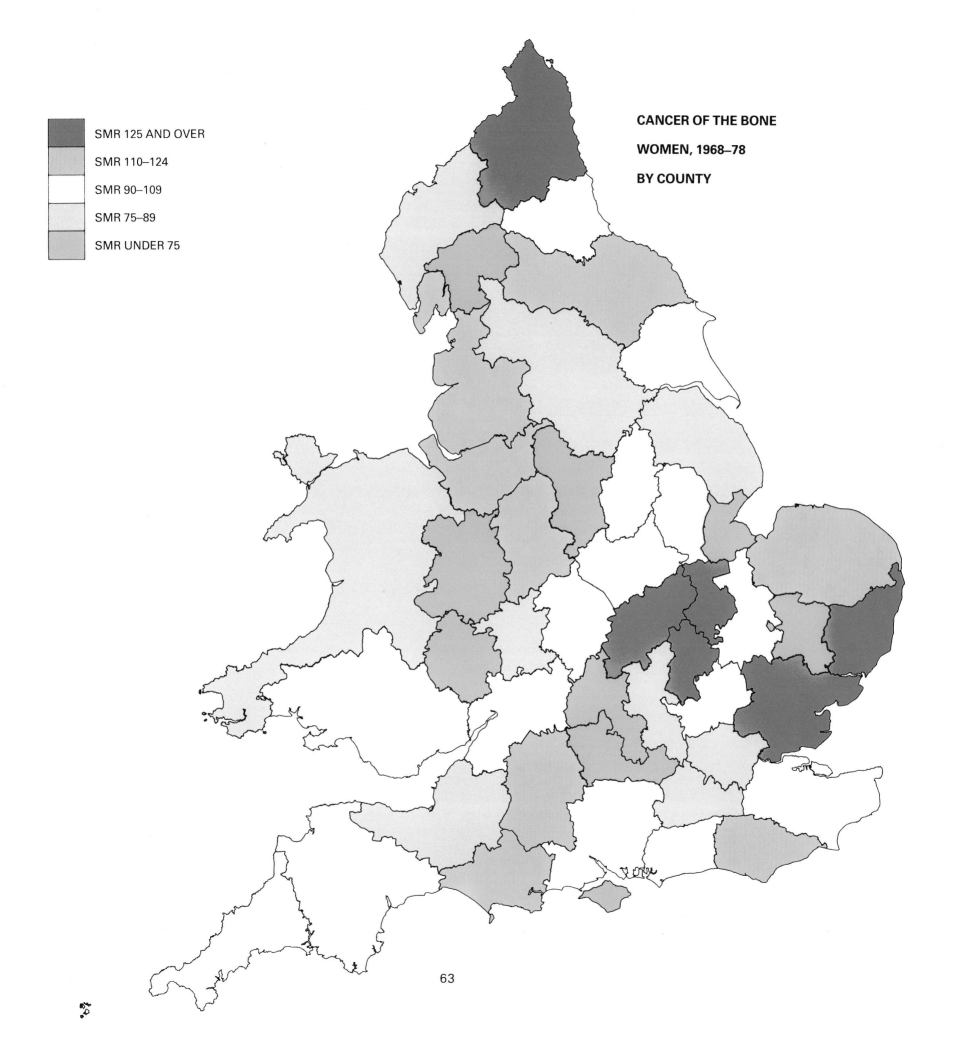

CANCER OF THE BONE

WOMEN, 1968–78

BY COUNTY

SMR 125 AND OVER

SMR 110–124

SMR 90–109

SMR 75–89

SMR UNDER 75

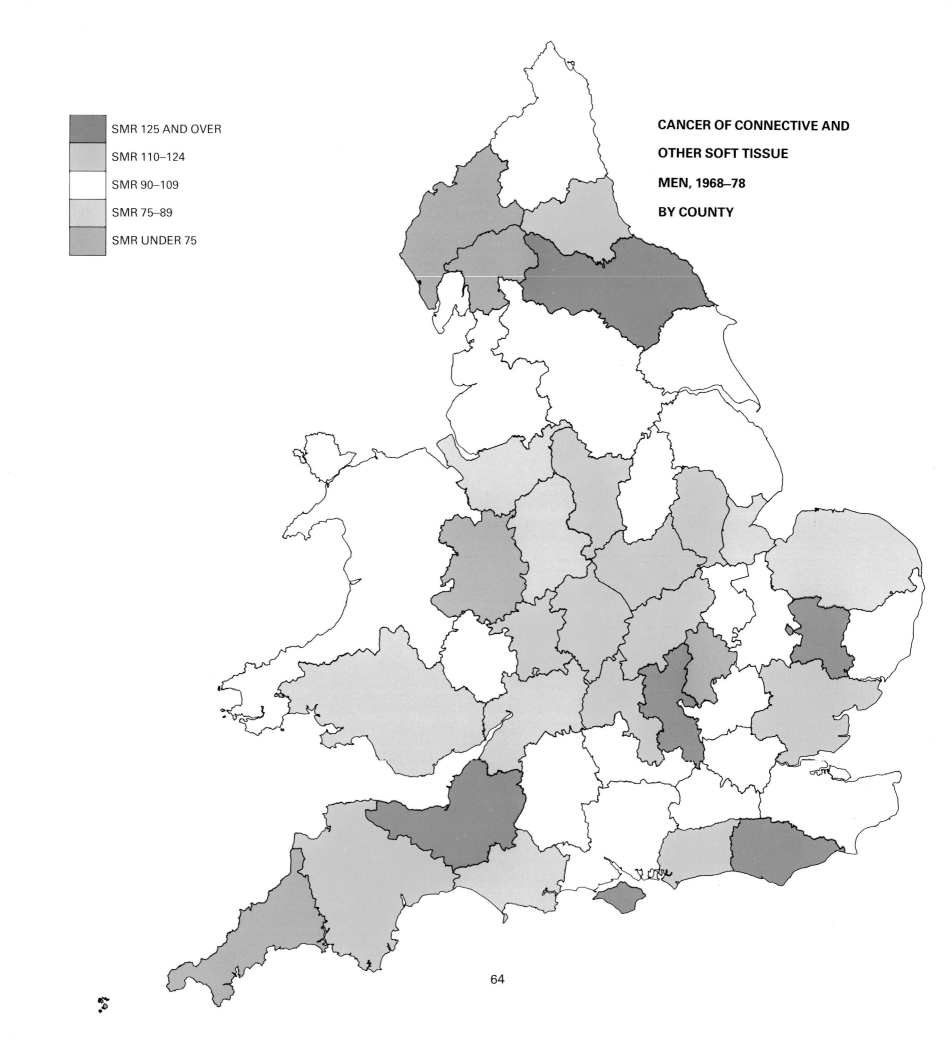

CANCER OF CONNECTIVE AND

OTHER SOFT TISSUE

MEN, 1968–78

BY COUNTY

SMR 125 AND OVER

SMR 110–124

SMR 90–109

SMR 75–89

SMR UNDER 75

64

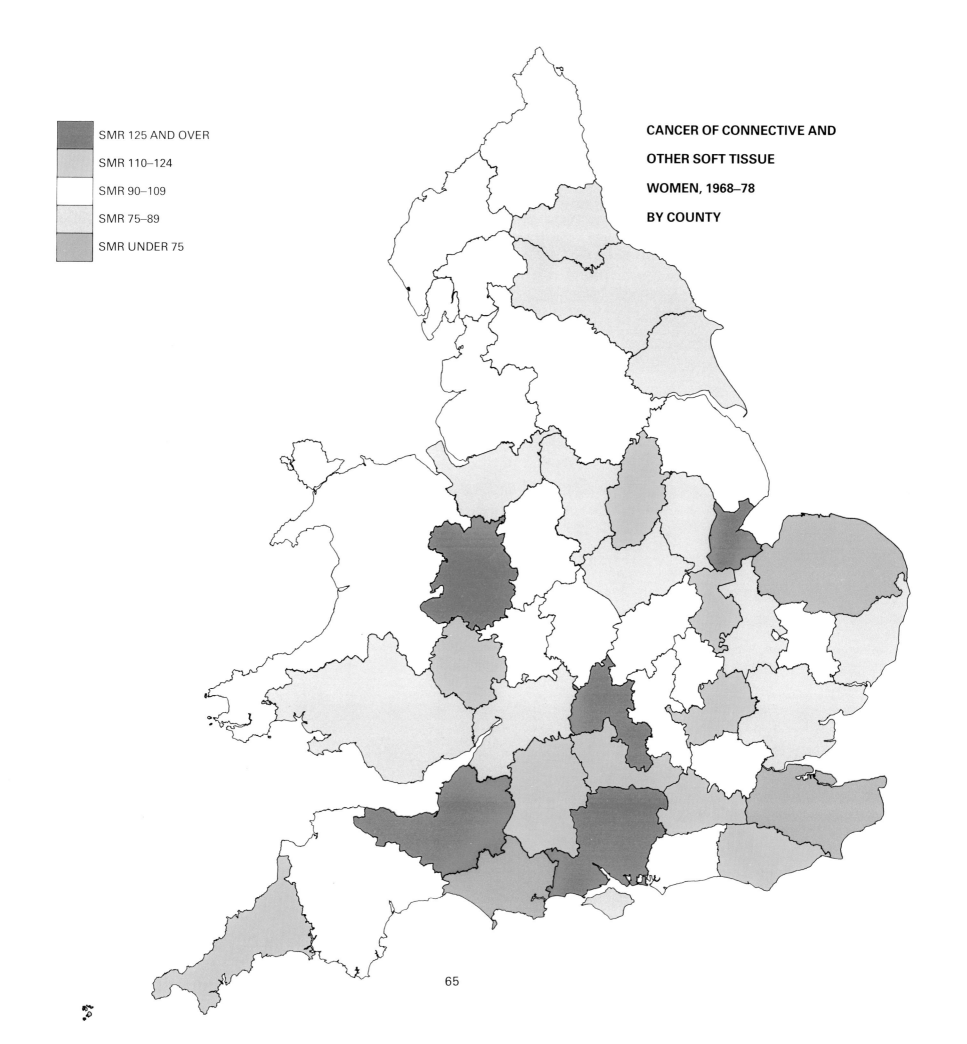

CANCER OF CONNECTIVE AND
OTHER SOFT TISSUE
WOMEN, 1968–78
BY COUNTY

SMR 125 AND OVER
SMR 110–124
SMR 90–109
SMR 75–89
SMR UNDER 75

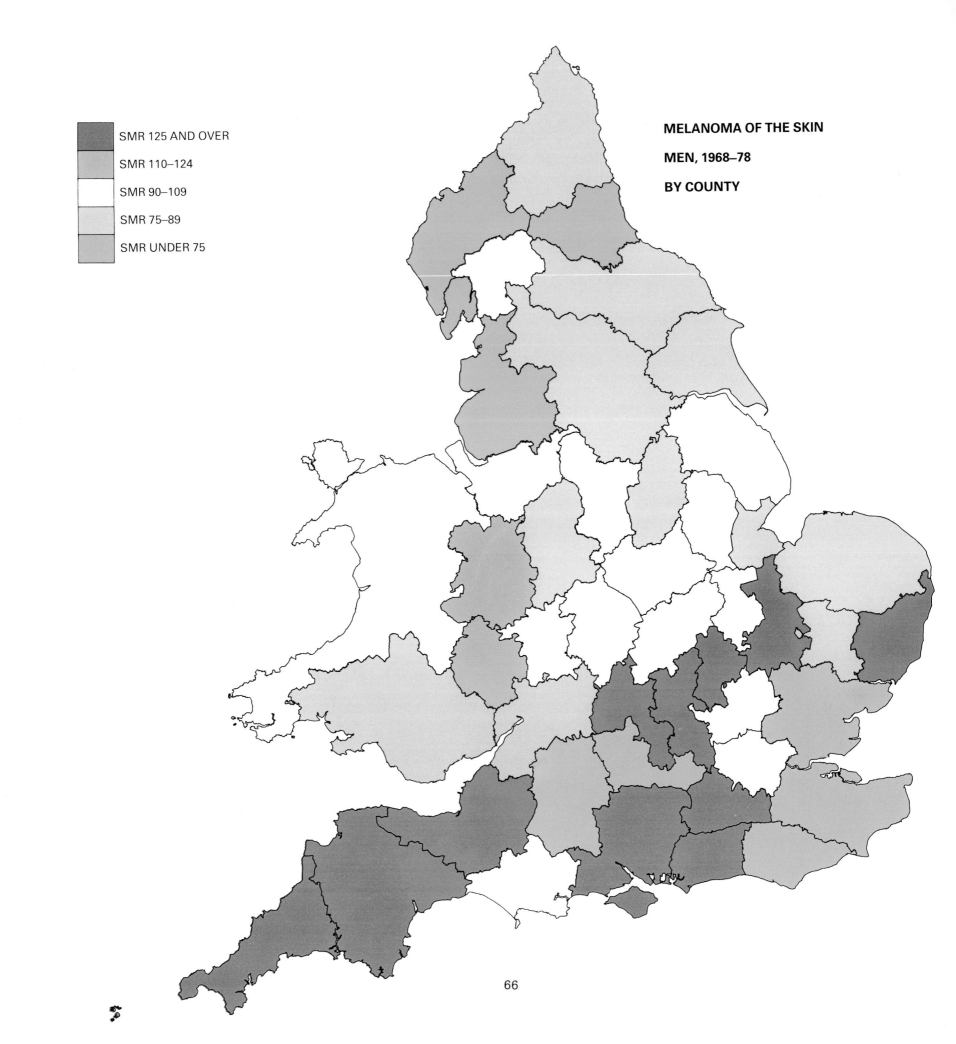

MELANOMA OF THE SKIN

MEN, 1968–78

BY COUNTY

SMR 125 AND OVER

SMR 110–124

SMR 90–109

SMR 75–89

SMR UNDER 75

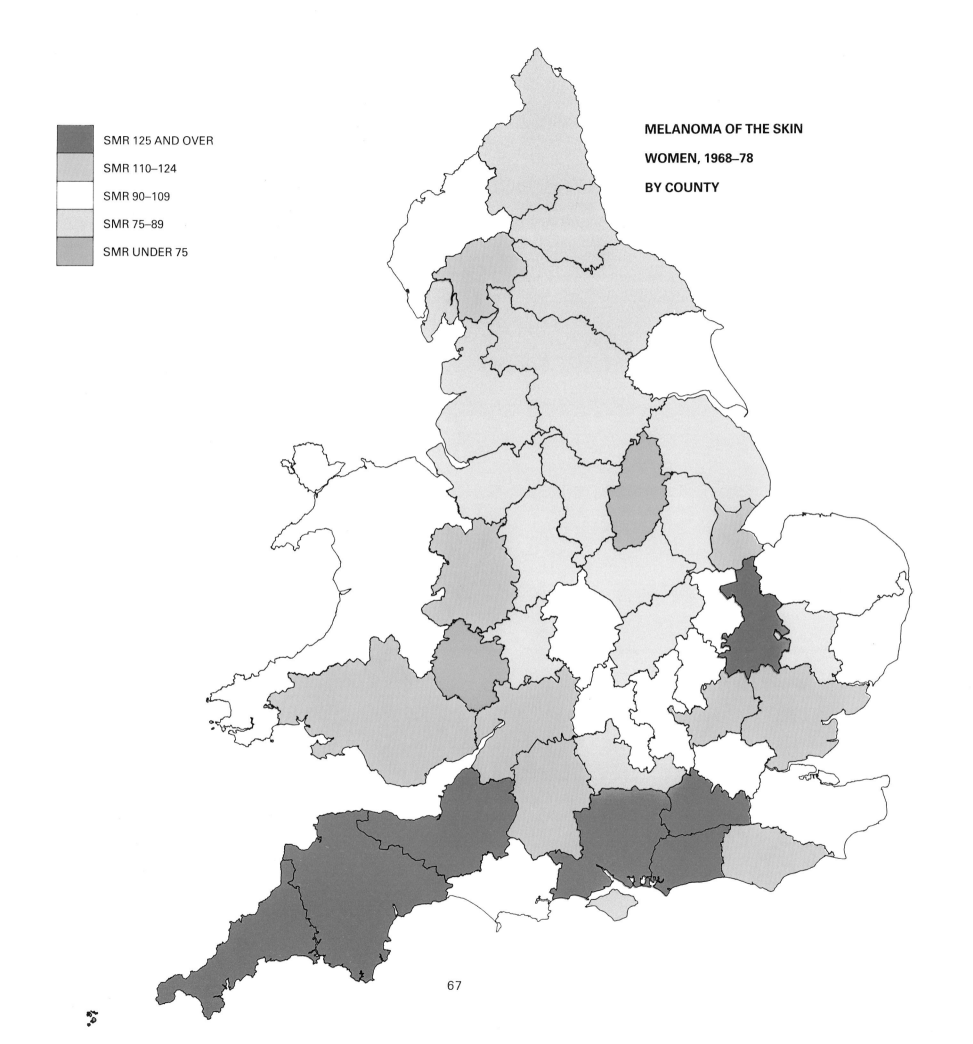

SMR 125 AND OVER

SMR 110–124

SMR 90–109

SMR 75–89

SMR UNDER 75

MELANOMA OF THE SKIN

WOMEN, 1968–78

BY COUNTY

67

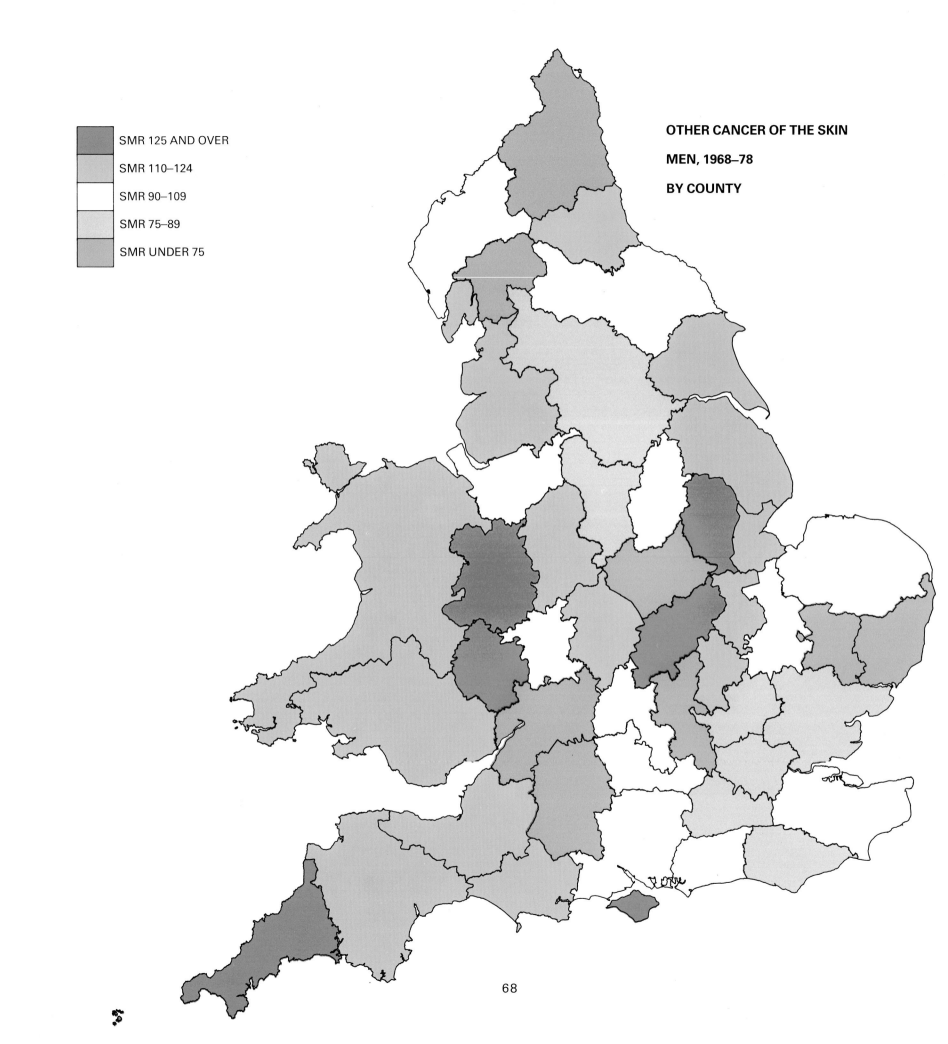

OTHER CANCER OF THE SKIN

MEN, 1968–78

BY COUNTY

SMR 125 AND OVER

SMR 110–124

SMR 90–109

SMR 75–89

SMR UNDER 75

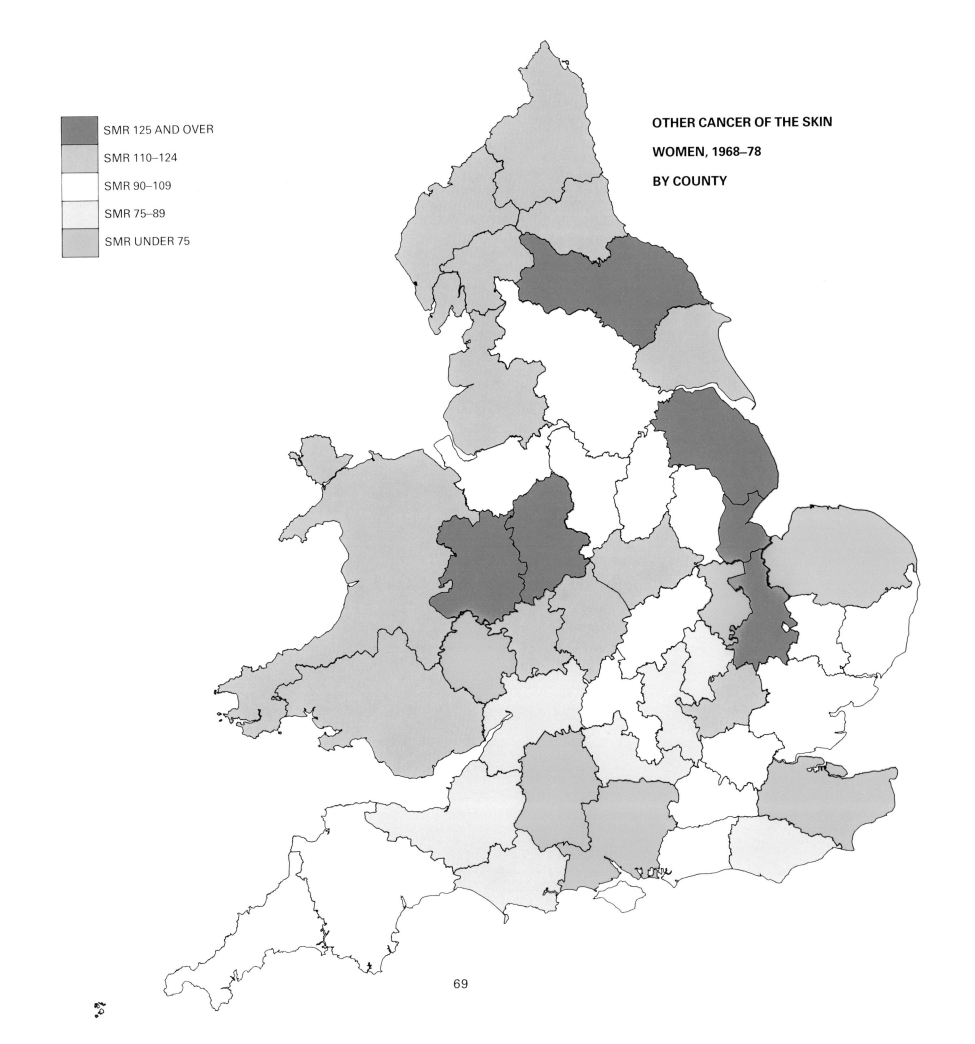

SMR 125 AND OVER

SMR 110–124

SMR 90–109

SMR 75–89

SMR UNDER 75

OTHER CANCER OF THE SKIN

WOMEN, 1968–78

BY COUNTY

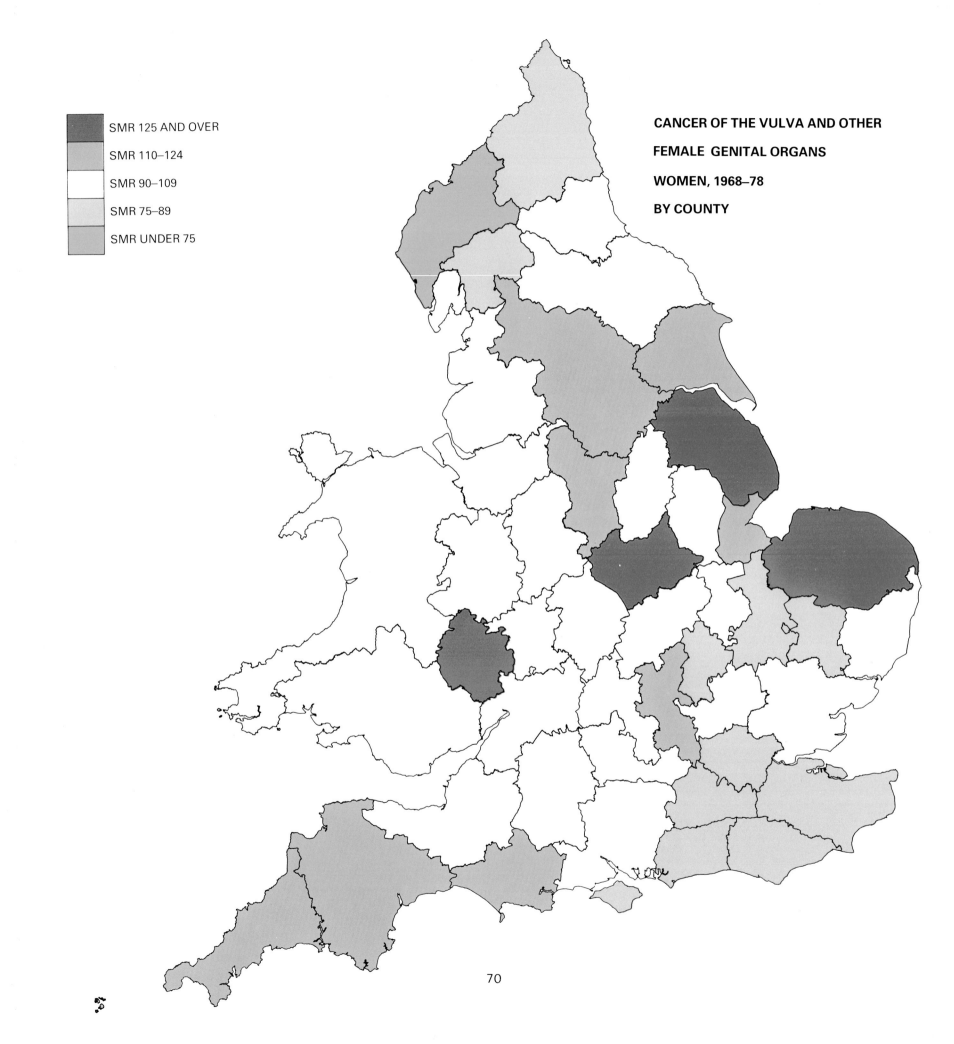

SMR 125 AND OVER

SMR 110–124

SMR 90–109

SMR 75–89

SMR UNDER 75

CANCER OF THE VULVA AND OTHER

FEMALE GENITAL ORGANS

WOMEN, 1968–78

BY COUNTY

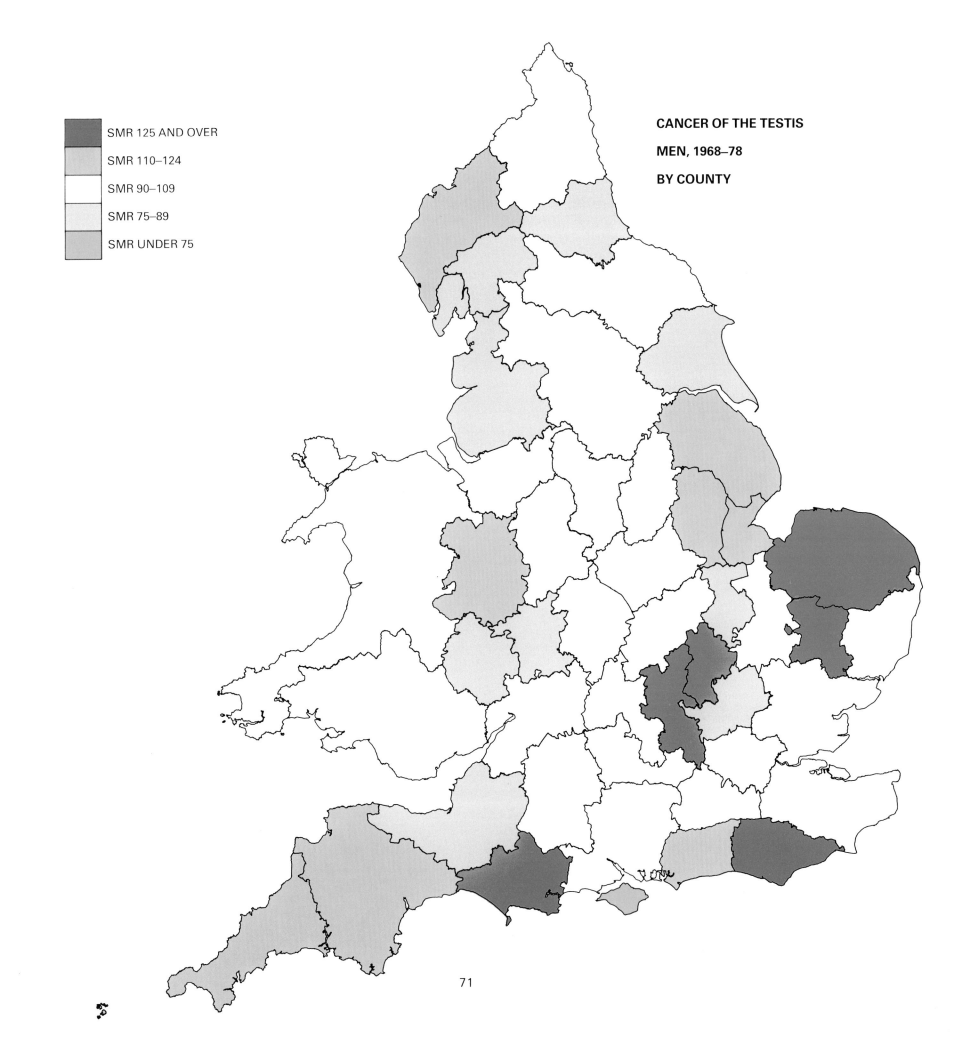

CANCER OF THE TESTIS

MEN, 1968–78

BY COUNTY

SMR 125 AND OVER

SMR 110–124

SMR 90–109

SMR 75–89

SMR UNDER 75

71

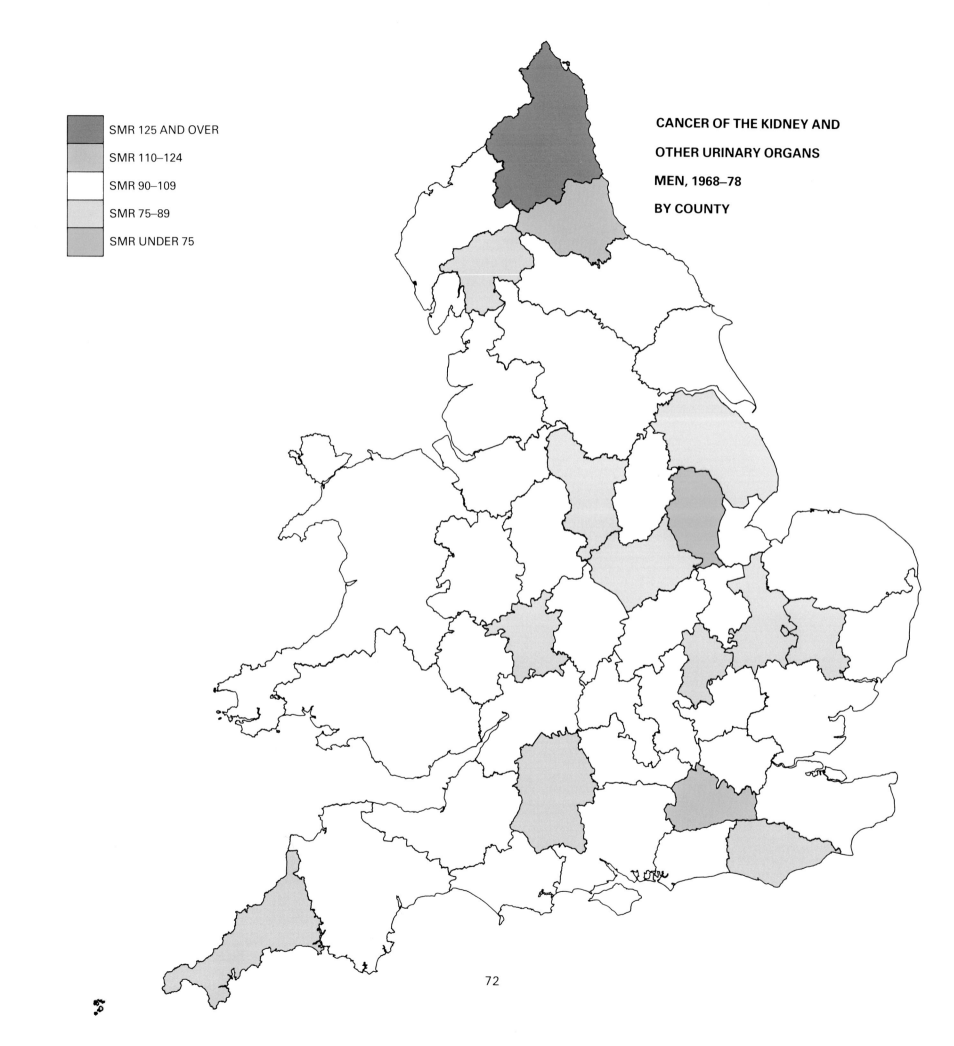

SMR 125 AND OVER

SMR 110–124

SMR 90–109

SMR 75–89

SMR UNDER 75

CANCER OF THE KIDNEY AND

OTHER URINARY ORGANS

MEN, 1968–78

BY COUNTY

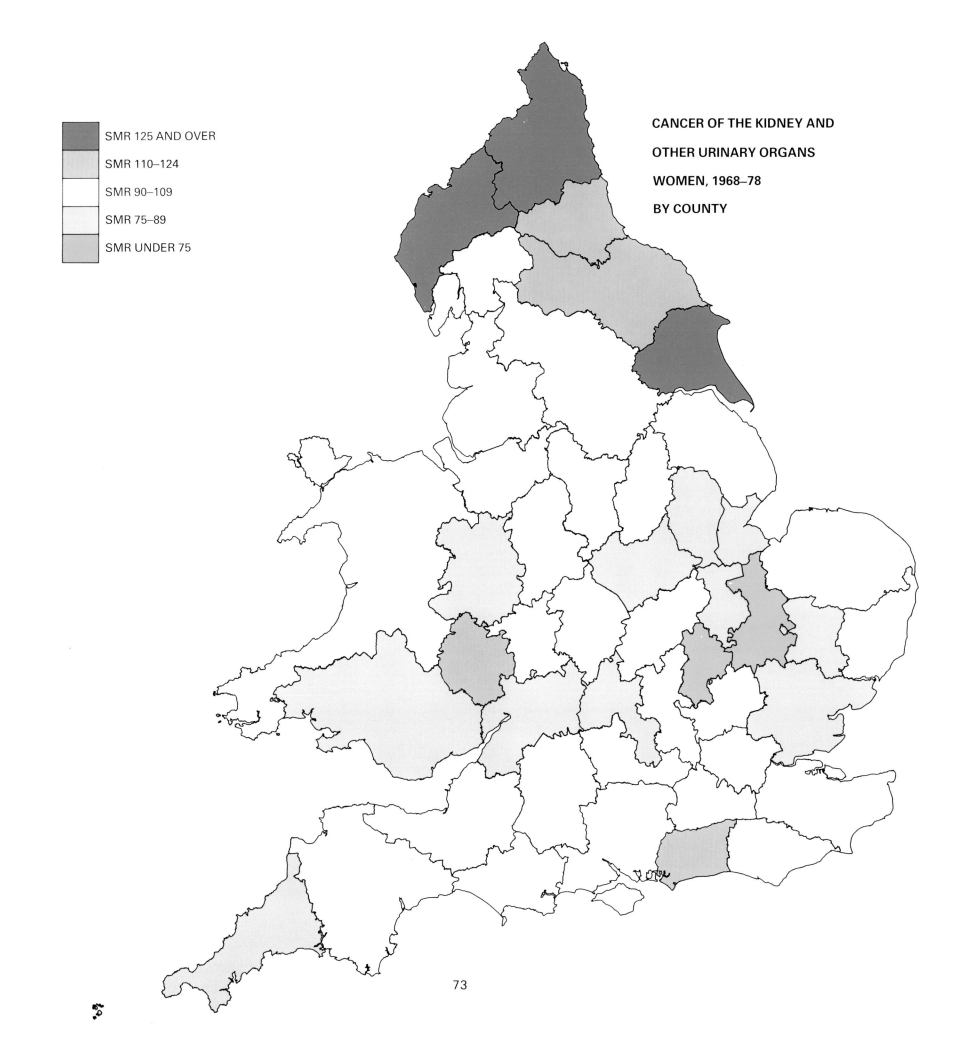

CANCER OF THE KIDNEY AND
OTHER URINARY ORGANS
WOMEN, 1968–78
BY COUNTY

SMR 125 AND OVER
SMR 110–124
SMR 90–109
SMR 75–89
SMR UNDER 75

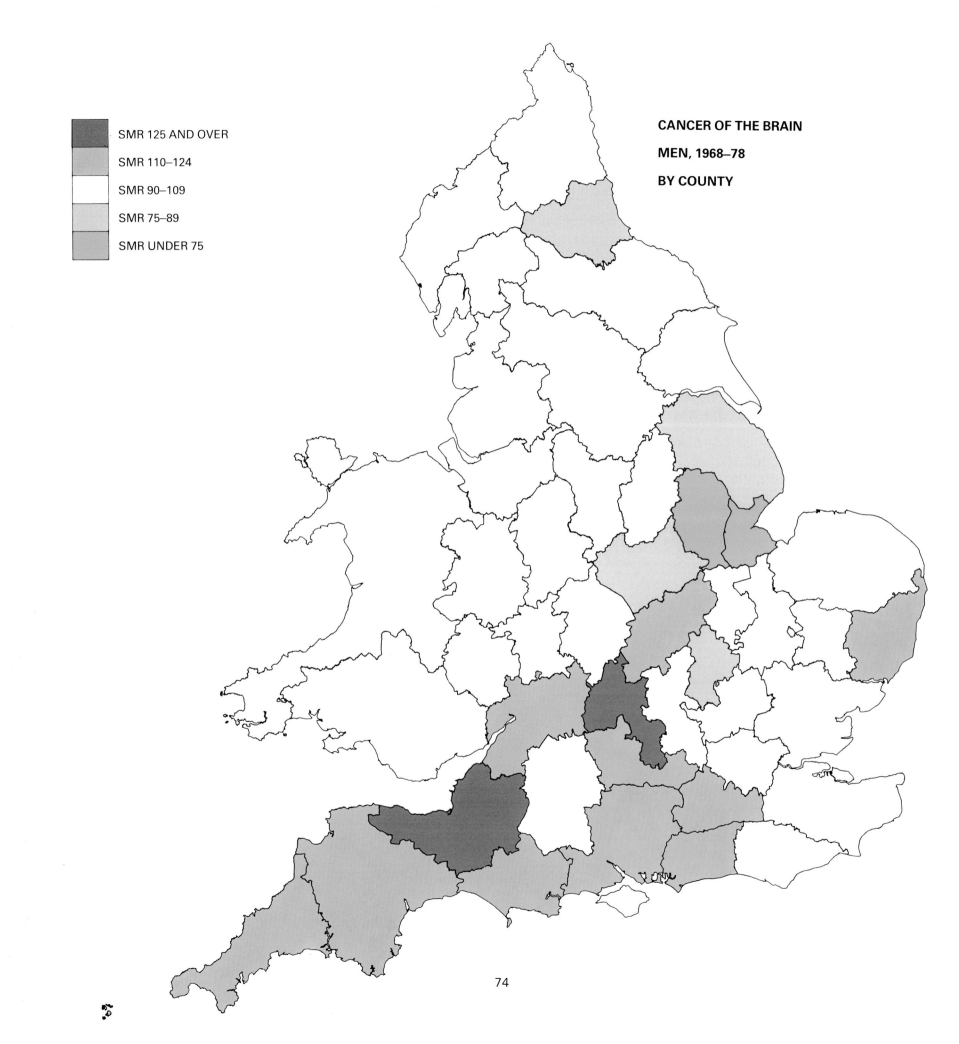

CANCER OF THE BRAIN

MEN, 1968–78

BY COUNTY

SMR 125 AND OVER

SMR 110–124

SMR 90–109

SMR 75–89

SMR UNDER 75

74

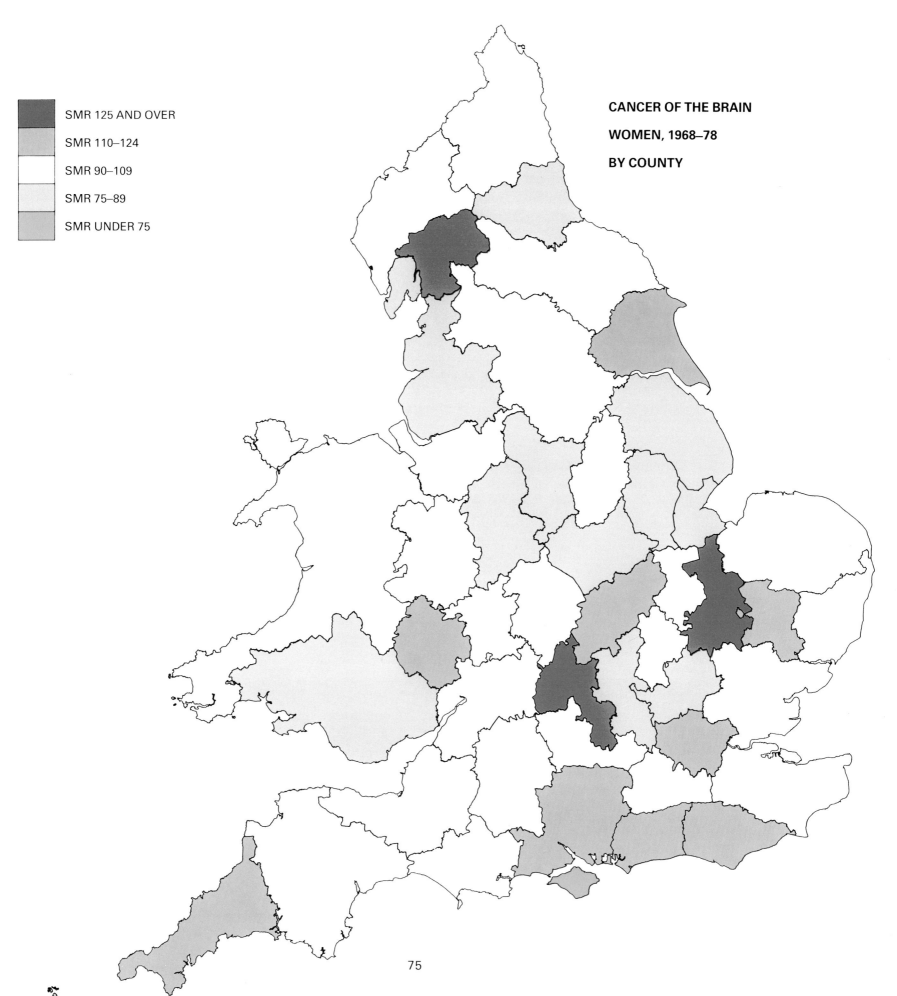

SMR 125 AND OVER

SMR 110–124

SMR 90–109

SMR 75–89

SMR UNDER 75

CANCER OF THE BRAIN

WOMEN, 1968–78

BY COUNTY

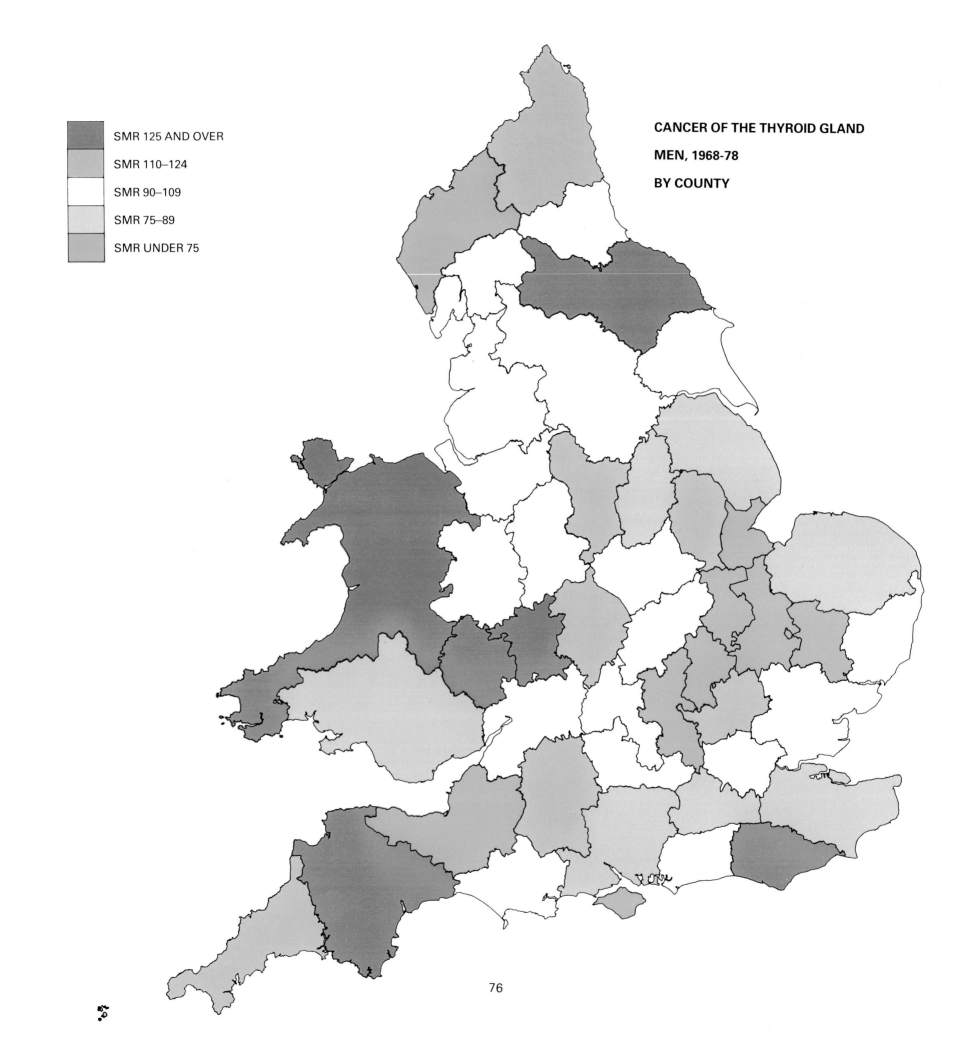

CANCER OF THE THYROID GLAND

MEN, 1968-78

BY COUNTY

SMR 125 AND OVER

SMR 110–124

SMR 90–109

SMR 75–89

SMR UNDER 75

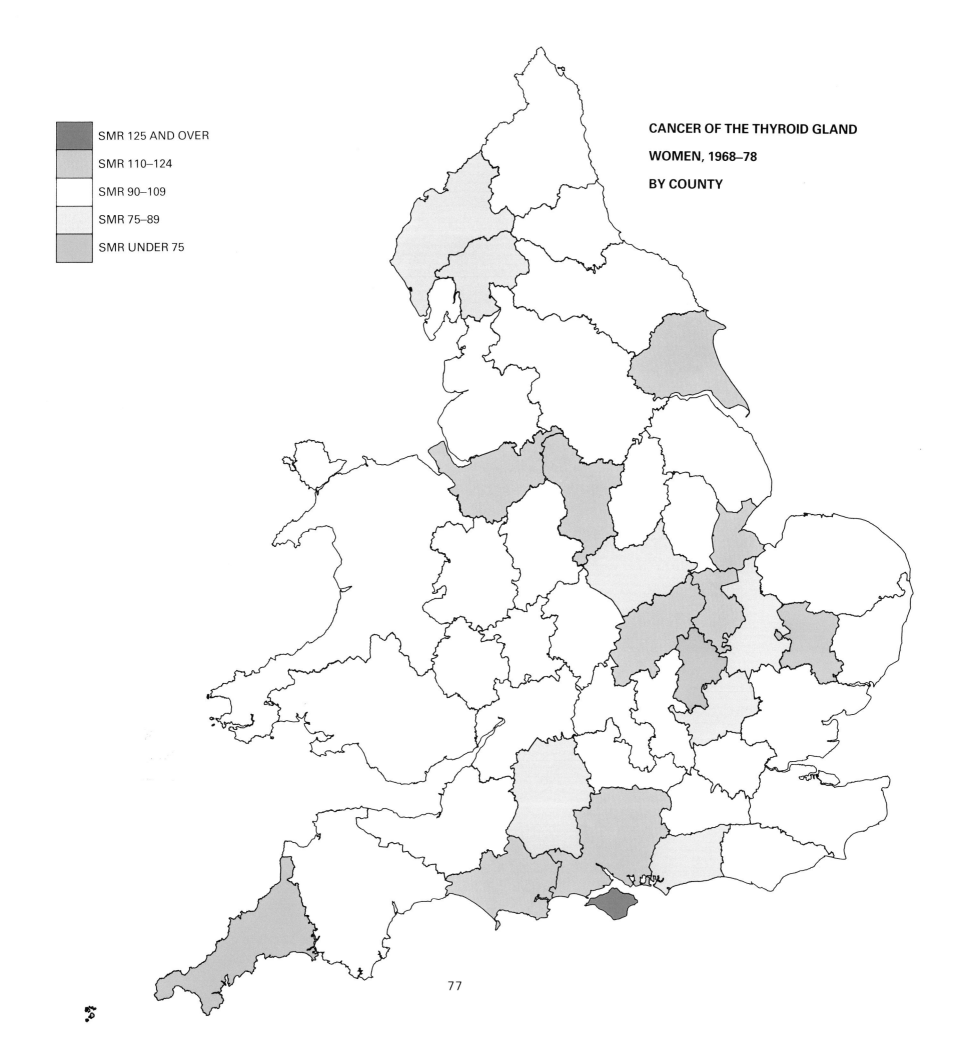

SMR 125 AND OVER

SMR 110–124

SMR 90–109

SMR 75–89

SMR UNDER 75

CANCER OF THE THYROID GLAND

WOMEN, 1968–78

BY COUNTY

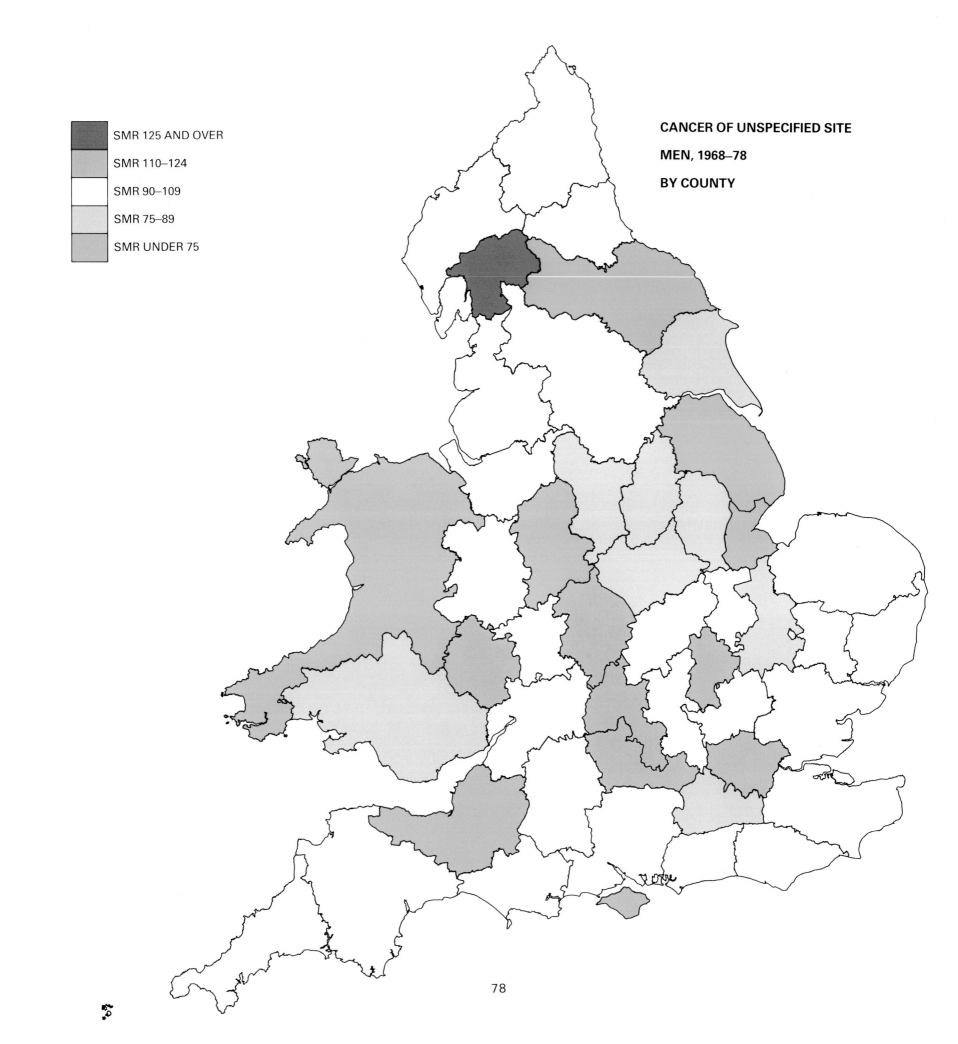

CANCER OF UNSPECIFIED SITE

MEN, 1968–78

BY COUNTY

SMR 125 AND OVER

SMR 110–124

SMR 90–109

SMR 75–89

SMR UNDER 75

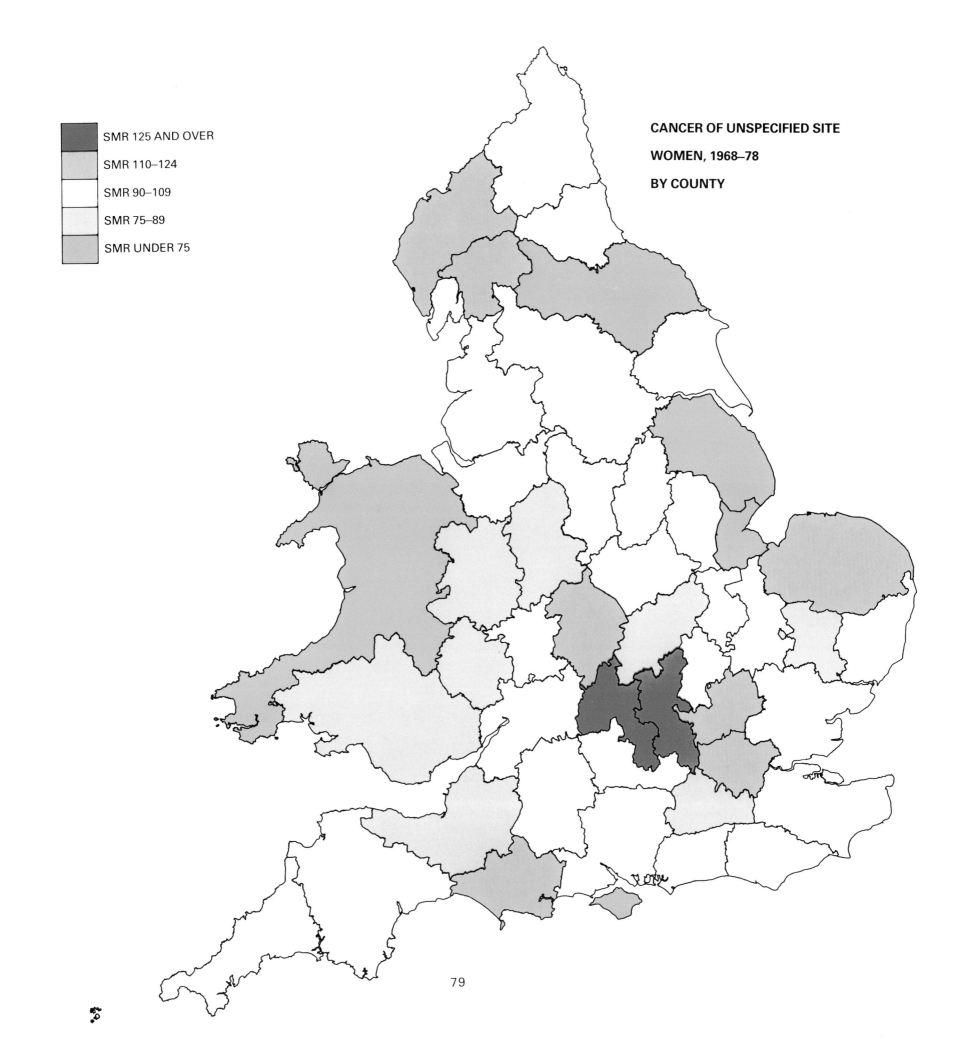

CANCER OF UNSPECIFIED SITE

WOMEN, 1968–78

BY COUNTY

SMR 125 AND OVER

SMR 110–124

SMR 90–109

SMR 75–89

SMR UNDER 75

79

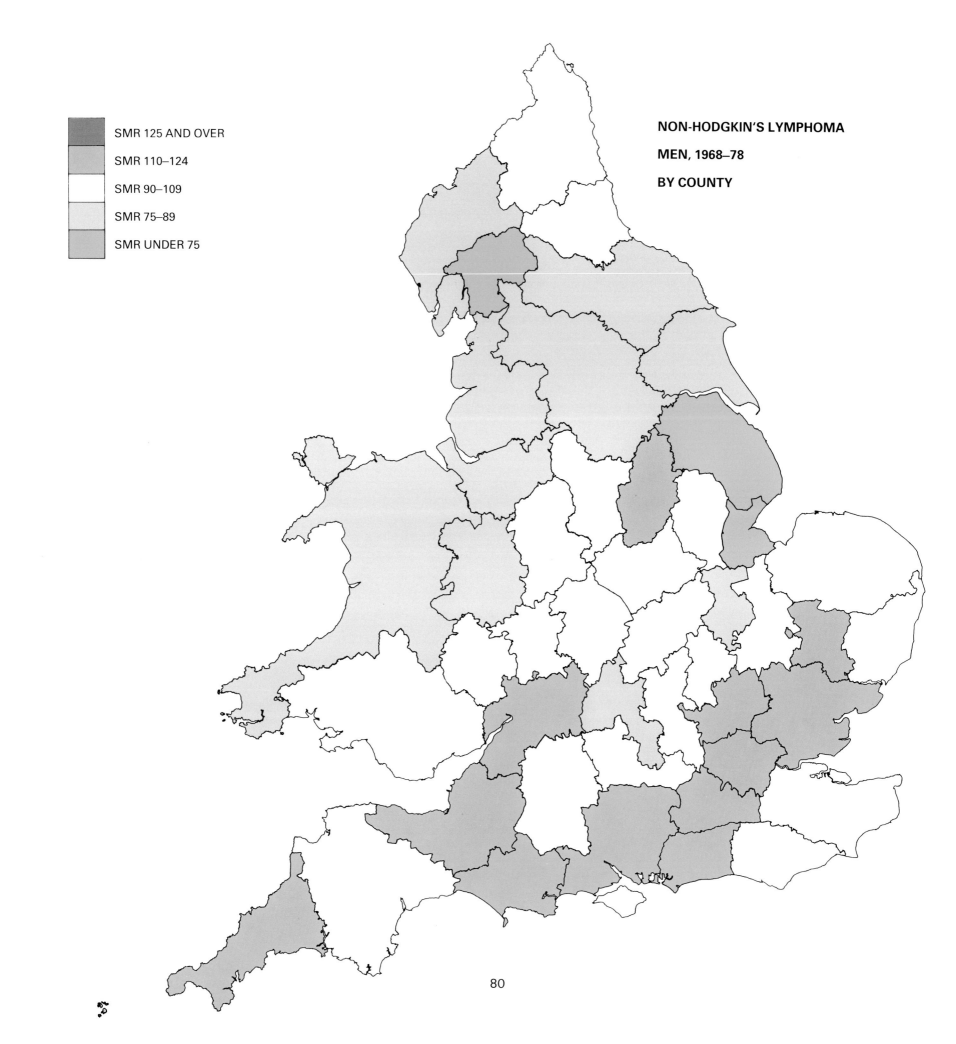

NON-HODGKIN'S LYMPHOMA

MEN, 1968–78

BY COUNTY

SMR 125 AND OVER

SMR 110–124

SMR 90–109

SMR 75–89

SMR UNDER 75

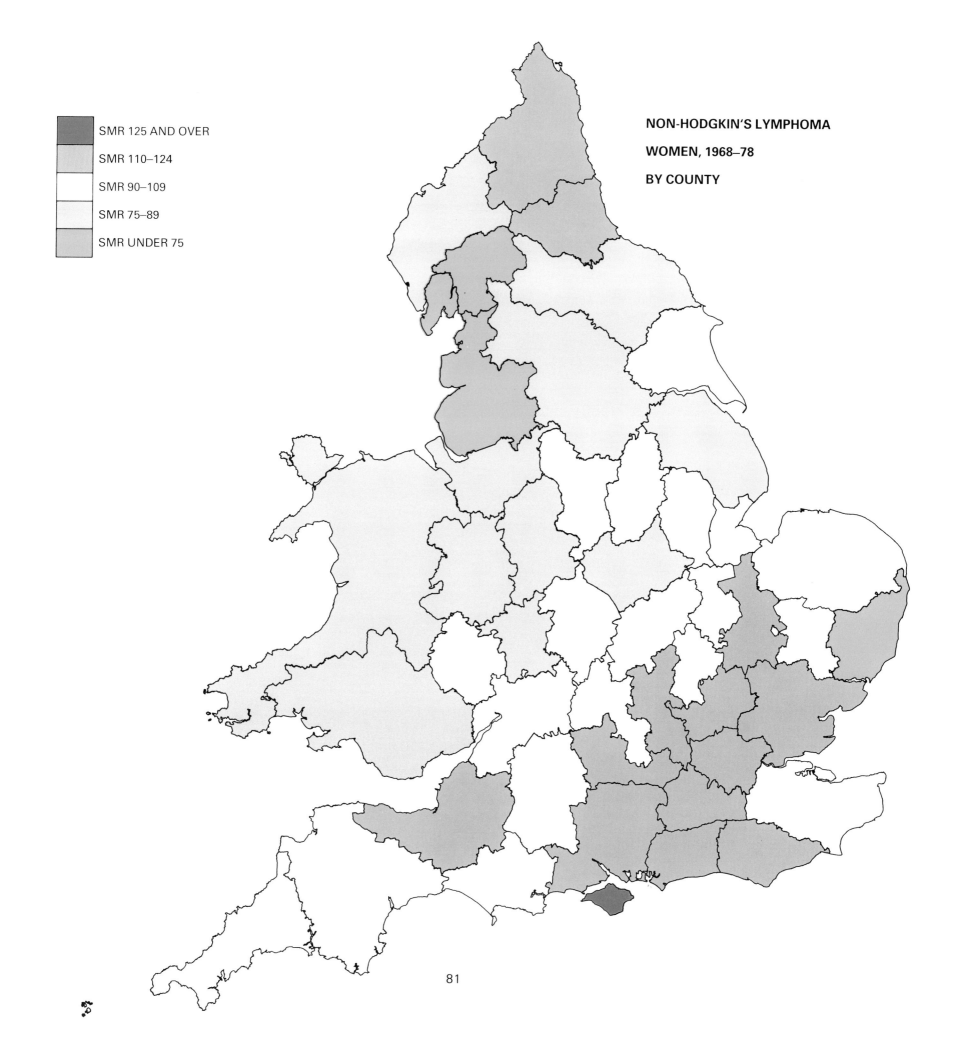

SMR 125 AND OVER

SMR 110–124

SMR 90–109

SMR 75–89

SMR UNDER 75

NON-HODGKIN'S LYMPHOMA

WOMEN, 1968–78

BY COUNTY

81

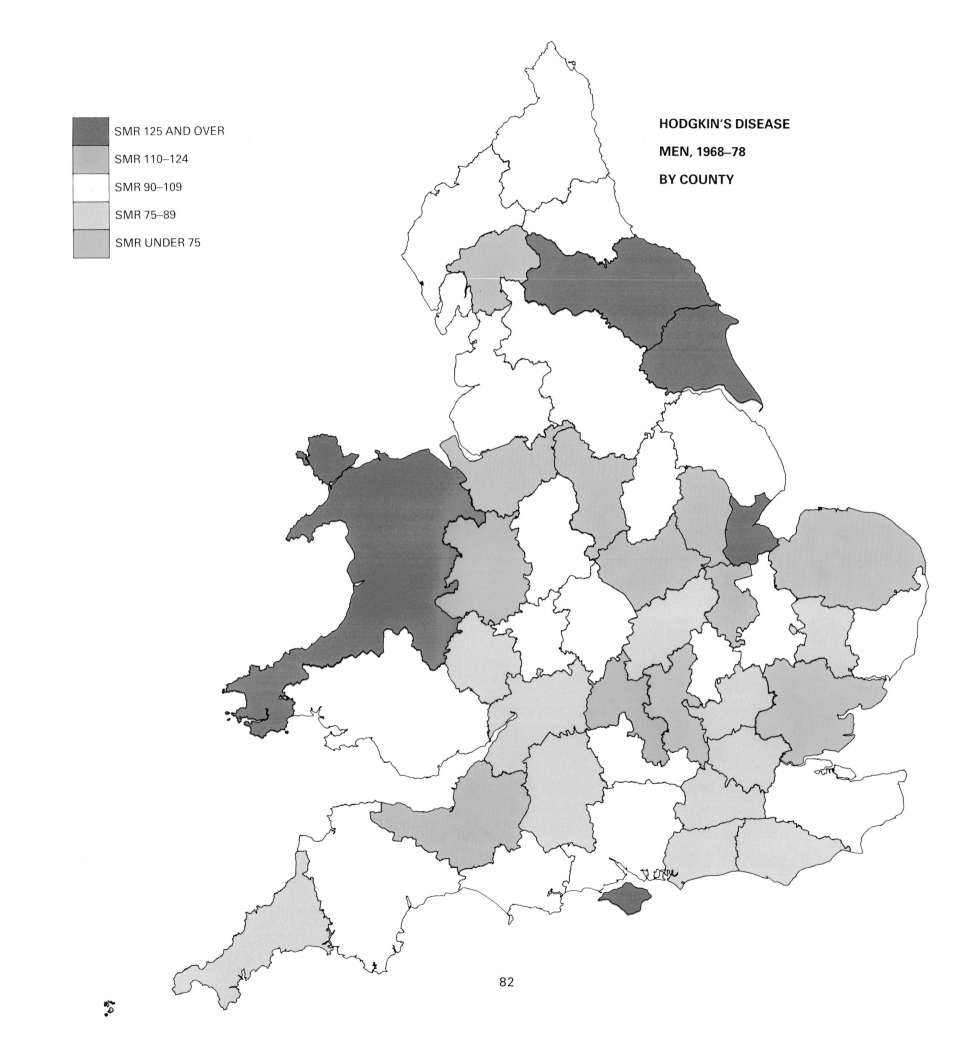

HODGKIN'S DISEASE

MEN, 1968–78

BY COUNTY

SMR 125 AND OVER

SMR 110–124

SMR 90–109

SMR 75–89

SMR UNDER 75

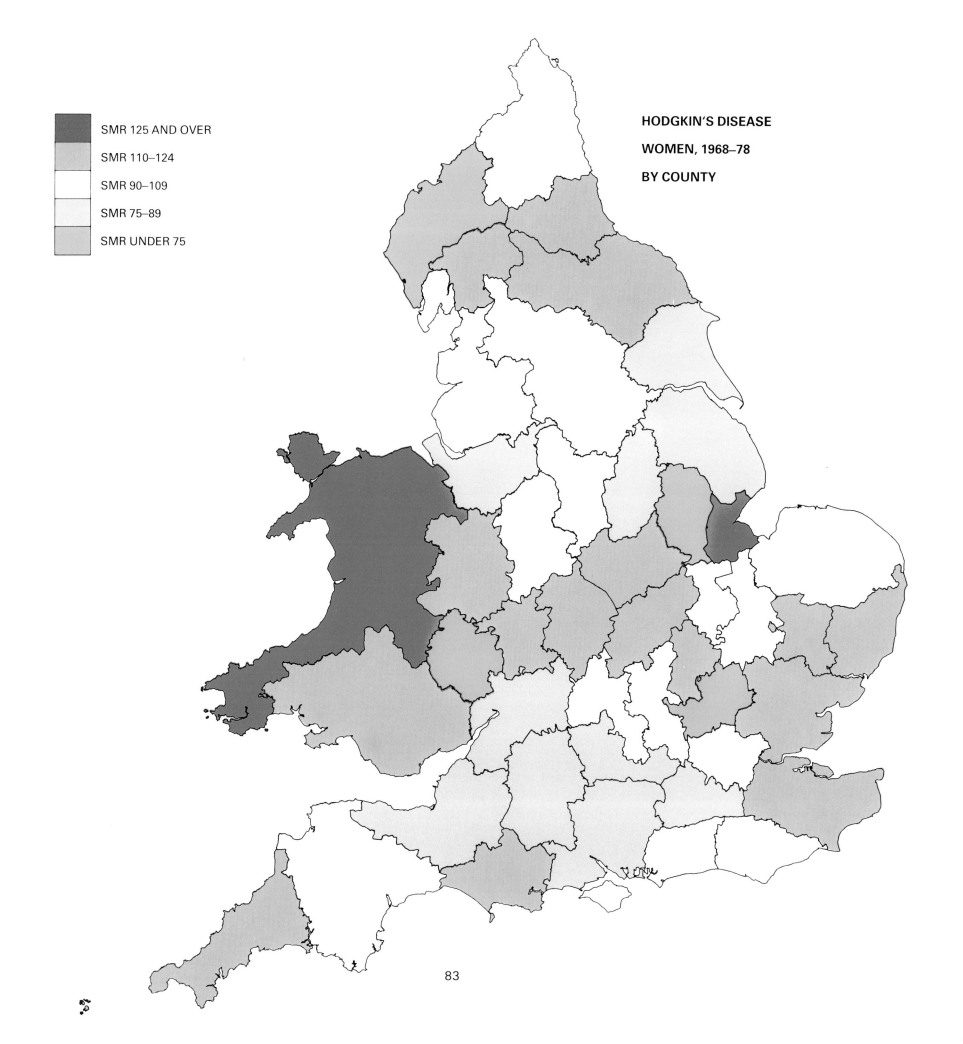

SMR 125 AND OVER

SMR 110–124

SMR 90–109

SMR 75–89

SMR UNDER 75

HODGKIN'S DISEASE

WOMEN, 1968–78

BY COUNTY

83

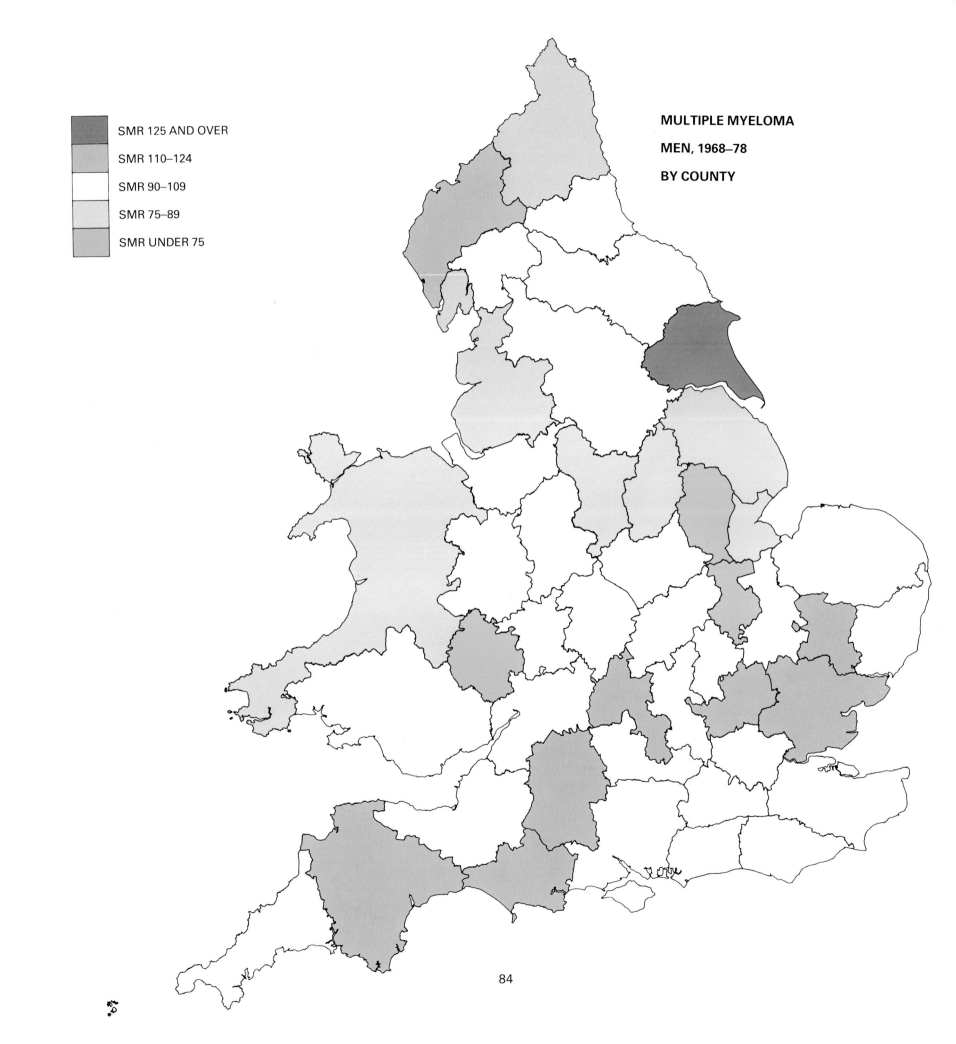

MULTIPLE MYELOMA

MEN, 1968–78

BY COUNTY

SMR 125 AND OVER

SMR 110–124

SMR 90–109

SMR 75–89

SMR UNDER 75

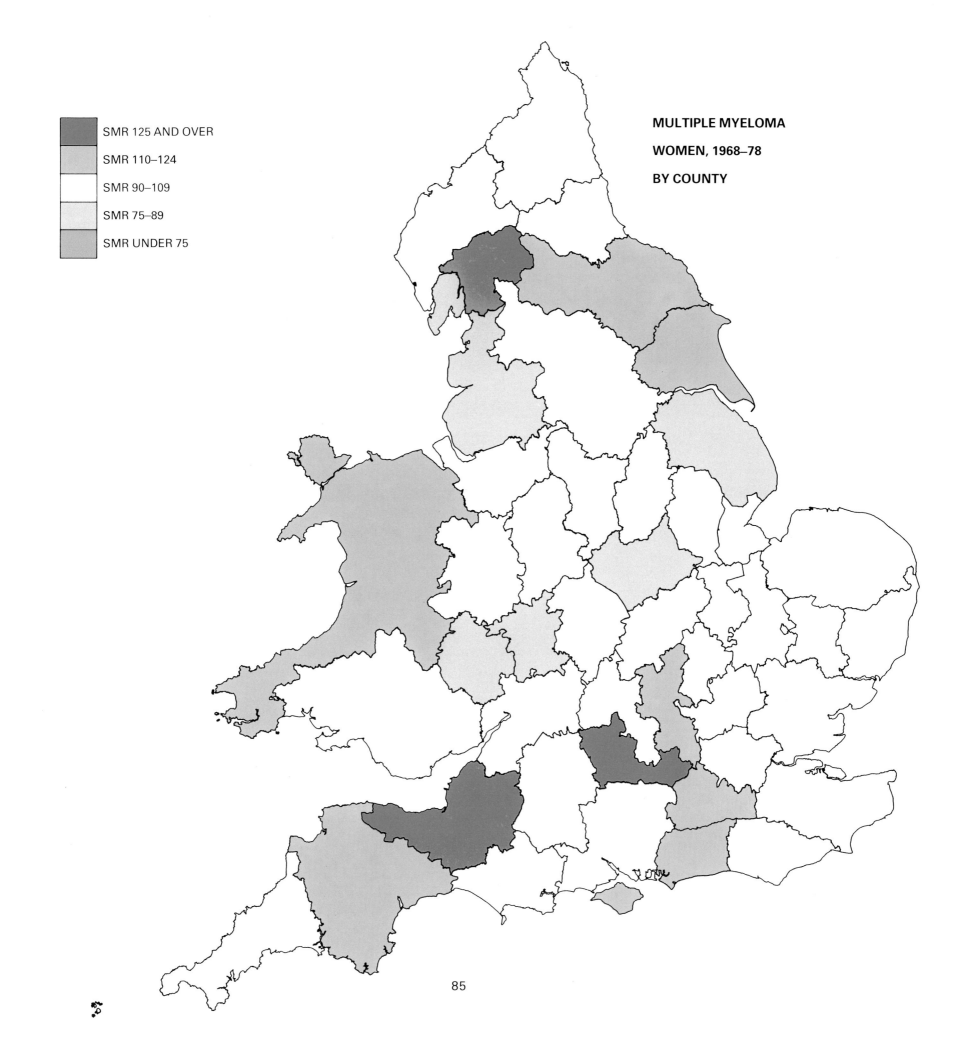

SMR 125 AND OVER

SMR 110–124

SMR 90–109

SMR 75–89

SMR UNDER 75

MULTIPLE MYELOMA

WOMEN, 1968–78

BY COUNTY

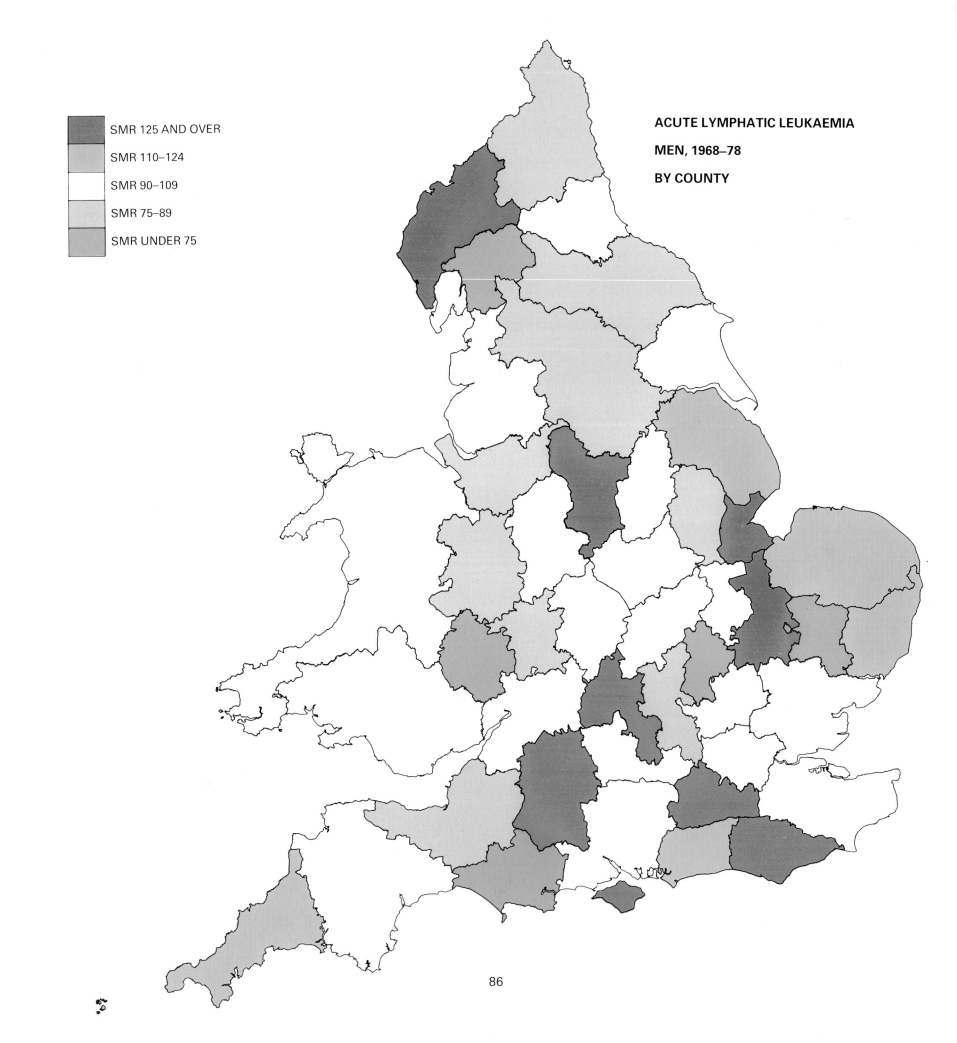

ACUTE LYMPHATIC LEUKAEMIA

MEN, 1968–78

BY COUNTY

SMR 125 AND OVER

SMR 110–124

SMR 90–109

SMR 75–89

SMR UNDER 75

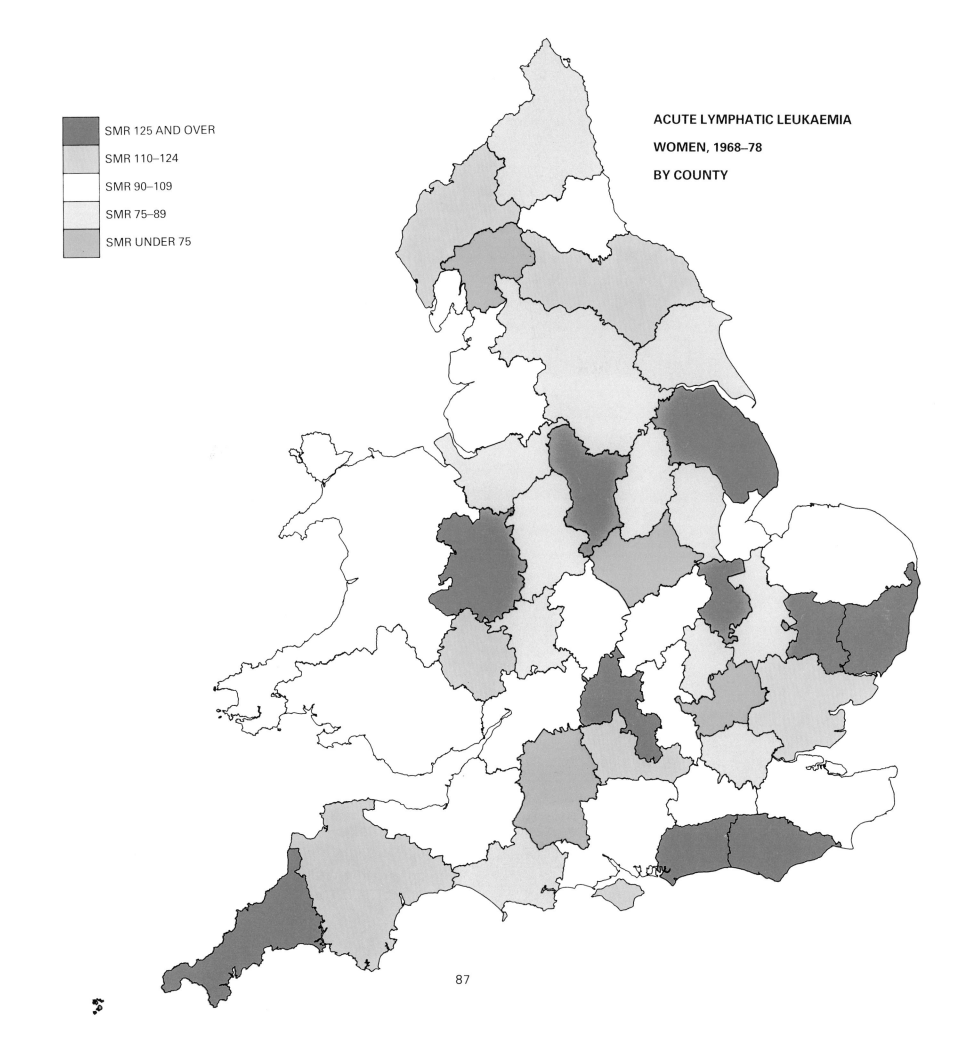

SMR 125 AND OVER

SMR 110–124

SMR 90–109

SMR 75–89

SMR UNDER 75

ACUTE LYMPHATIC LEUKAEMIA

WOMEN, 1968–78

BY COUNTY

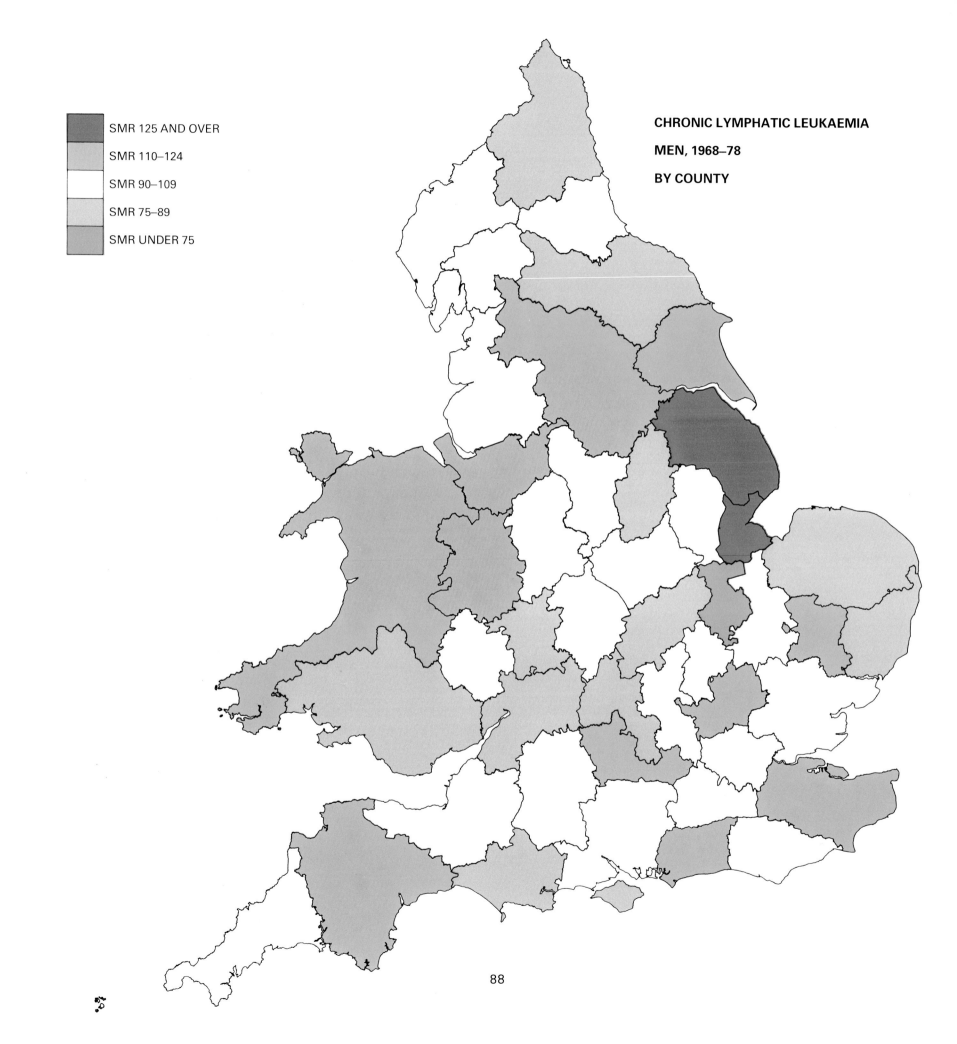

CHRONIC LYMPHATIC LEUKAEMIA

MEN, 1968–78

BY COUNTY

SMR 125 AND OVER

SMR 110–124

SMR 90–109

SMR 75–89

SMR UNDER 75

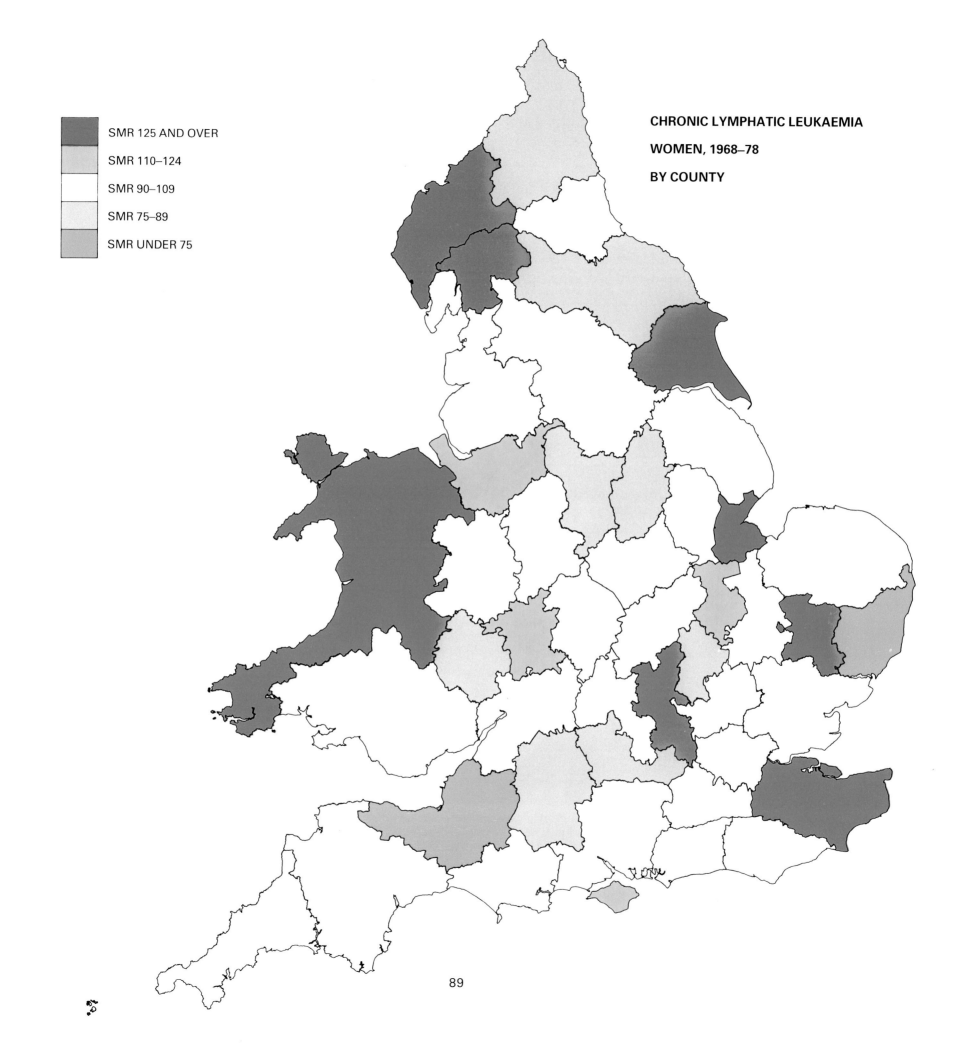

CHRONIC LYMPHATIC LEUKAEMIA

WOMEN, 1968–78

BY COUNTY

SMR 125 AND OVER

SMR 110–124

SMR 90–109

SMR 75–89

SMR UNDER 75

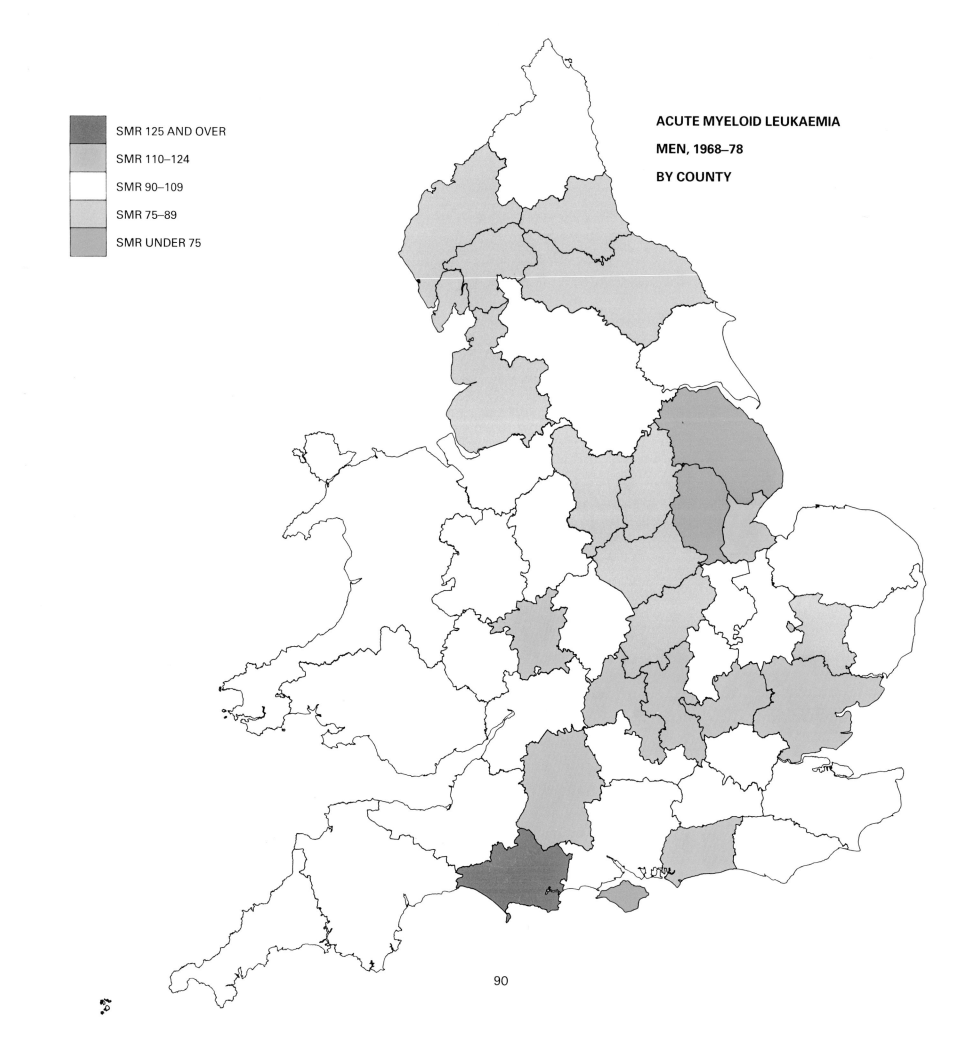

SMR 125 AND OVER

SMR 110–124

SMR 90–109

SMR 75–89

SMR UNDER 75

ACUTE MYELOID LEUKAEMIA

MEN, 1968–78

BY COUNTY

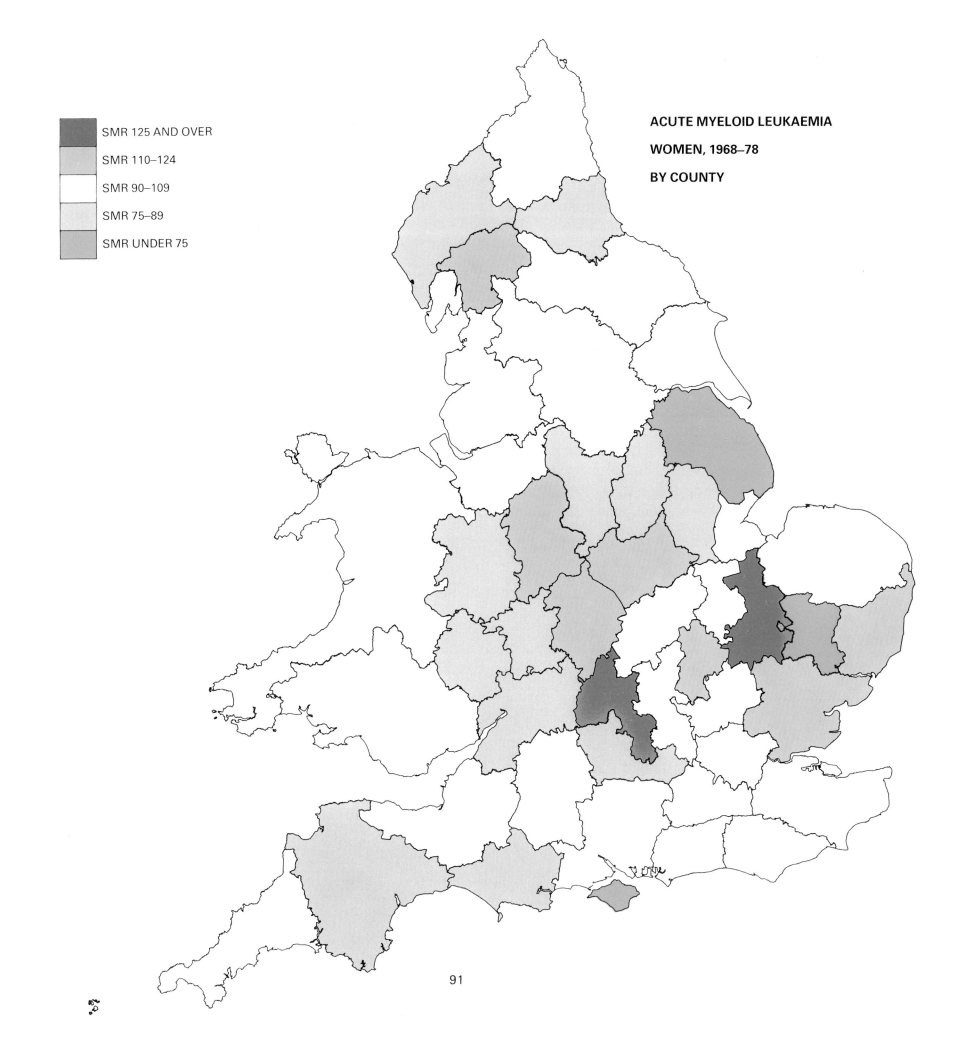

ACUTE MYELOID LEUKAEMIA

WOMEN, 1968–78

BY COUNTY

SMR 125 AND OVER

SMR 110–124

SMR 90–109

SMR 75–89

SMR UNDER 75

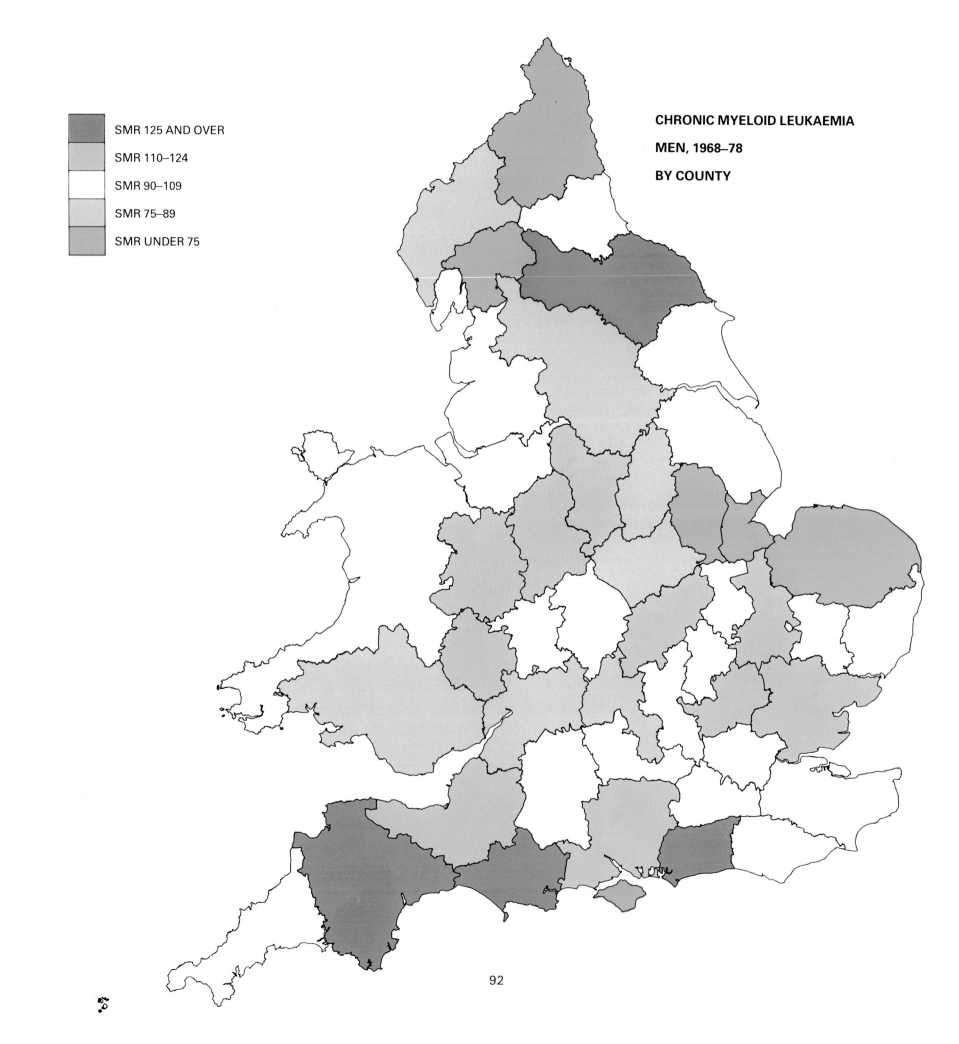

CHRONIC MYELOID LEUKAEMIA

MEN, 1968–78

BY COUNTY

SMR 125 AND OVER

SMR 110–124

SMR 90–109

SMR 75–89

SMR UNDER 75

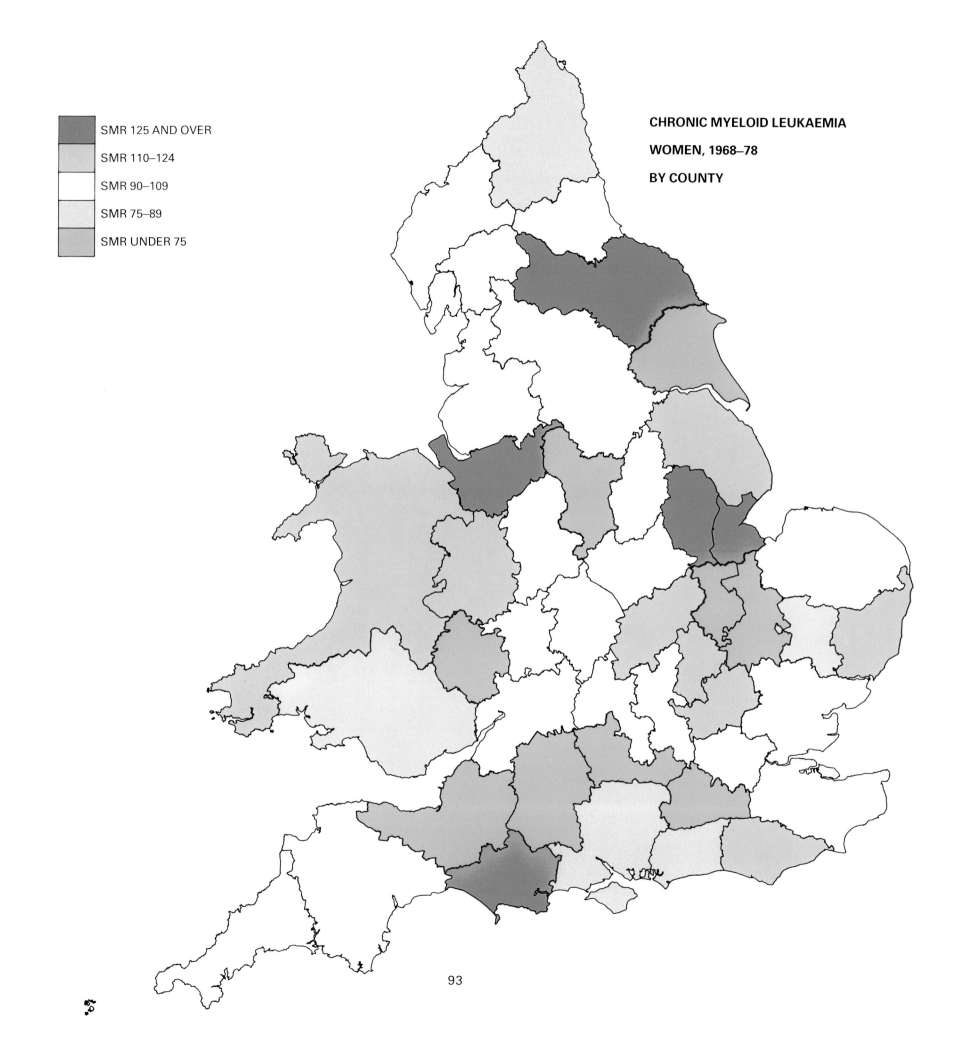

SMR 125 AND OVER

SMR 110–124

SMR 90–109

SMR 75–89

SMR UNDER 75

CHRONIC MYELOID LEUKAEMIA

WOMEN, 1968–78

BY COUNTY

MORTALITY FROM CANCER OF THE BUCCAL CAVITY
IN ENGLAND AND WALES DURING 1968–78

NUMBER OF DEATHS DURING 1968–78 AND AVERAGE ANNUAL DEATH RATES PER MILLION BY SEX AND AGE GROUPS

AGE GROUP (YEARS)	MEN		WOMEN	
	NUMBER OF DEATHS	RATE PER MILLION	NUMBER OF DEATHS	RATE PER MILLION
0	1	0.2	0	0.0
1–4	2	0.1	3	0.2
5–14	6	0.1	4	0.1
15–24	10	0.3	9	0.2
25–34	42	1	28	1
35–44	120	4	85	3
45–54	519	16	268	8
55–64	1,211	40	577	17
65–74	1,878	97	973	37
75+	2,057	254	1,572	90
ALL AGES	5,846	22	3,519	13

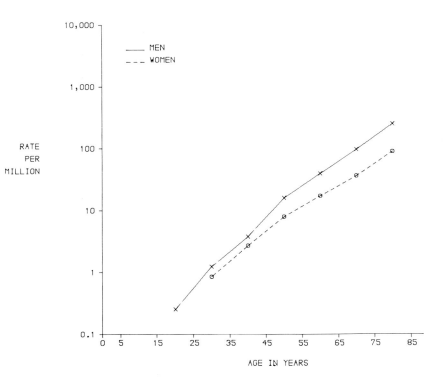

NUMBER OF THE 47 'COUNTY' AREAS SHOWN ON MAP BY LEVEL OF THE STANDARDISED MORTALITY RATIO (SMR) DURING 1968–78

STANDARDISED MORTALITY RATIO	NUMBER OF AREAS	
	MEN	WOMEN
125 AND OVER	4	6
110–124	6	5
90–109	18	17
75–89	11	10
UNDER 75	8	9
LOWEST SMR	59.9	61.3
HIGHEST SMR	165.2	184.8
NUMBER OF AREAS WITH ZERO DEATHS	0	0

MORTALITY FROM CANCER OF THE PHARYNX
IN ENGLAND AND WALES DURING 1968–78

NUMBER OF DEATHS DURING 1968–78 AND AVERAGE ANNUAL
DEATH RATES PER MILLION BY SEX AND AGE GROUPS

AGE GROUP (YEARS)	MEN		WOMEN	
	NUMBER OF DEATHS	RATE PER MILLION	NUMBER OF DEATHS	RATE PER MILLION
0	0	0.0	0	0.0
1–4	2	0.1	4	0.2
5–14	13	0.3	7	0.2
15–24	29	1	19	0.5
25–34	41	1	30	1
35–44	116	4	111	4
45–54	489	15	438	13
55–64	1,222	40	779	23
65–74	1,633	85	1,042	39
75+	1,204	149	914	53
ALL AGES	4,749	18	3,344	12

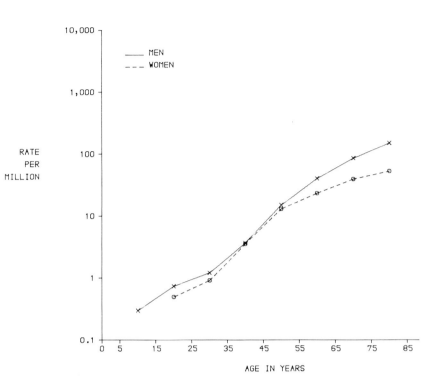

NUMBER OF THE 47 'COUNTY' AREAS SHOWN ON MAP BY LEVEL OF
THE STANDARDISED MORTALITY RATIO (SMR) DURING 1968–78

STANDARDISED MORTALITY RATIO	NUMBER OF AREAS	
	MEN	WOMEN
125 AND OVER	2	8
110–124	8	5
90–109	19	11
75–89	10	12
UNDER 75	8	11
LOWEST SMR	24.9	35.1
HIGHEST SMR	193.6	156.1
NUMBER OF AREAS WITH ZERO DEATHS	0	0

MORTALITY FROM CANCER OF THE LIVER
IN ENGLAND AND WALES DURING 1968–78

NUMBER OF DEATHS DURING 1968–78 AND AVERAGE ANNUAL
DEATH RATES PER MILLION BY SEX AND AGE GROUPS

AGE GROUP (YEARS)	MEN		WOMEN	
	NUMBER OF DEATHS	RATE PER MILLION	NUMBER OF DEATHS	RATE PER MILLION
0	11	3	11	3
1–4	26	1	20	1
5–14	13	0.3	15	0.4
15–24	35	1	30	1
25–34	55	2	38	1
35–44	131	4	80	3
45–54	466	14	225	7
55–64	1,104	36	399	12
65–74	1,203	62	660	25
75+	629	78	699	40
ALL AGES	3,673	14	2,177	8

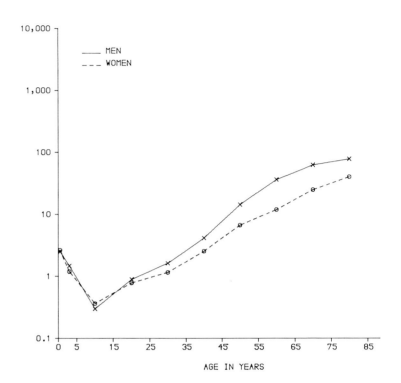

NUMBER OF THE 47 'COUNTY' AREAS SHOWN ON MAP BY LEVEL OF
THE STANDARDISED MORTALITY RATIO (SMR) DURING 1968–78

STANDARDISED MORTALITY RATIO	NUMBER OF AREAS	
	MEN	WOMEN
125 AND OVER	3	6
110–124	6	5
90–109	17	17
75–89	11	9
UNDER 75	10	10
LOWEST SMR	41.3	15.7
HIGHEST SMR	134.3	200.1
NUMBER OF AREAS WITH ZERO DEATHS	0	0

MORTALITY FROM CANCER OF THE GALL BLADDER
IN ENGLAND AND WALES DURING 1968–78

NUMBER OF DEATHS DURING 1968–78 AND AVERAGE ANNUAL
DEATH RATES PER MILLION BY SEX AND AGE GROUPS

AGE GROUP (YEARS)	MEN		WOMEN	
	NUMBER OF DEATHS	RATE PER MILLION	NUMBER OF DEATHS	RATE PER MILLION
0	0	0.0	0	0.0
1–4	1	0.1	2	0.1
5–14	1	0.0	0	0.0
15–24	3	0.1	3	0.1
25–34	28	1	19	1
35–44	100	3	91	3
45–54	382	12	432	13
55–64	1,134	37	1,239	37
65–74	1,717	89	2,731	102
75+	1,159	143	3,104	178
ALL AGES	4,525	17	7,621	28

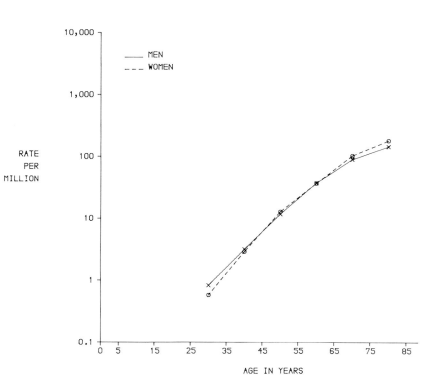

NUMBER OF THE 47 'COUNTY' AREAS SHOWN ON MAP BY LEVEL OF
THE STANDARDISED MORTALITY RATIO (SMR) DURING 1968–78

STANDARDISED MORTALITY RATIO	NUMBER OF AREAS	
	MEN	WOMEN
125 AND OVER	1	3
110–124	7	8
90–109	18	23
75–89	14	10
UNDER 75	7	3
LOWEST SMR	38.8	68.1
HIGHEST SMR	125.6	138.0
NUMBER OF AREAS WITH ZERO DEATHS	0	0

MORTALITY FROM CANCER OF THE NOSE
IN ENGLAND AND WALES DURING 1968–78

NUMBER OF DEATHS DURING 1968–78 AND AVERAGE ANNUAL
DEATH RATES PER MILLION BY SEX AND AGE GROUPS

AGE GROUP (YEARS)	MEN		WOMEN	
	NUMBER OF DEATHS	RATE PER MILLION	NUMBER OF DEATHS	RATE PER MILLION
0	0	0.0	1	0.2
1–4	4	0.2	3	0.2
5–14	15	0.3	10	0.2
15–24	13	0.3	8	0.2
25–34	22	1	16	0.5
35–44	64	2	33	1
45–54	210	6	123	4
55–64	412	14	235	7
65–74	502	26	360	14
75+	322	40	427	25
ALL AGES	1,564	6	1,216	4

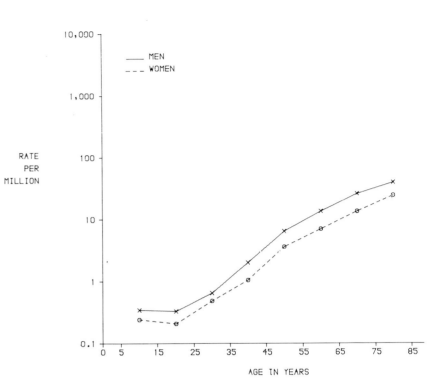

NUMBER OF THE 47 'COUNTY' AREAS SHOWN ON MAP BY LEVEL OF
THE STANDARDISED MORTALITY RATIO (SMR) DURING 1968–78

STANDARDISED MORTALITY RATIO	NUMBER OF AREAS	
	MEN	WOMEN
125 AND OVER	5	11
110–124	9	4
90–109	16	14
75–89	9	7
UNDER 75	8	11
LOWEST SMR	26.3	28.1
HIGHEST SMR	205.2	228.8
NUMBER OF AREAS WITH ZERO DEATHS	0	0

MORTALITY FROM CANCER OF THE LARYNX
IN ENGLAND AND WALES DURING 1968–78

NUMBER OF DEATHS DURING 1968–78 AND AVERAGE ANNUAL
DEATH RATES PER MILLION BY SEX AND AGE GROUPS

AGE GROUP (YEARS)	MEN		WOMEN	
	NUMBER OF DEATHS	RATE PER MILLION	NUMBER OF DEATHS	RATE PER MILLION
0	0	0.0	0	0.0
1–4	0	0.0	0	0.0
5–14	0	0.0	0	0.0
15–24	2	0.1	2	0.1
25–34	12	0.4	7	0.2
35–44	107	3	26	1
45–54	565	17	166	5
55–64	1,569	52	419	12
65–74	2,546	132	497	19
75+	1,839	227	432	25
ALL AGES	6,640	25	1,549	6

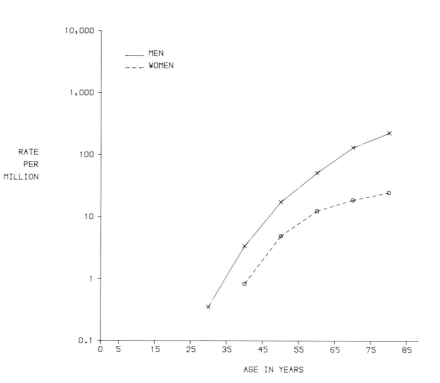

NUMBER OF THE 47 'COUNTY' AREAS SHOWN ON MAP BY LEVEL OF
THE STANDARDISED MORTALITY RATIO (SMR) DURING 1968–78

STANDARDISED MORTALITY RATIO	NUMBER OF AREAS	
	MEN	WOMEN
125 AND OVER	0	6
110–124	7	4
90–109	21	19
75–89	13	6
UNDER 75	6	12
LOWEST SMR	61.1	0.0
HIGHEST SMR	122.0	169.7
NUMBER OF AREAS WITH ZERO DEATHS	0	1

MORTALITY FROM CANCER OF THE BONE
IN ENGLAND AND WALES DURING 1968–78

NUMBER OF DEATHS DURING 1968–78 AND AVERAGE ANNUAL DEATH RATES PER MILLION BY SEX AND AGE GROUPS

AGE GROUP (YEARS)	MEN		WOMEN	
	NUMBER OF DEATHS	RATE PER MILLION	NUMBER OF DEATHS	RATE PER MILLION
0	1	0.2	4	1
1–4	12	1	18	1
5–14	188	4	154	4
15–24	355	9	223	6
25–34	135	4	85	3
35–44	137	4	80	3
45–54	305	9	166	5
55–64	543	18	347	10
65–74	784	41	582	22
75+	547	68	692	40
ALL AGES	3,007	12	2,351	9

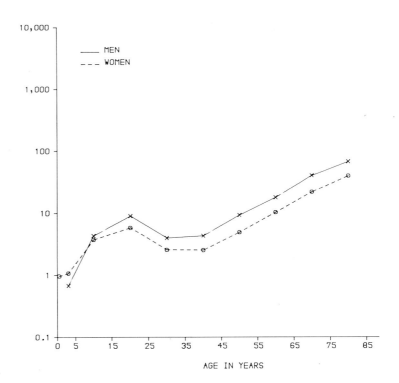

NUMBER OF THE 47 'COUNTY' AREAS SHOWN ON MAP BY LEVEL OF THE STANDARDISED MORTALITY RATIO (SMR) DURING 1968–78

STANDARDISED MORTALITY RATIO	NUMBER OF AREAS	
	MEN	WOMEN
125 AND OVER	1	6
110–124	6	8
90–109	21	15
75–89	12	9
UNDER 75	7	9
LOWEST SMR	20.8	19.8
HIGHEST SMR	137.6	145.4
NUMBER OF AREAS WITH ZERO DEATHS	0	0

MORTALITY FROM CANCER OF CONNECTIVE AND OTHER SOFT TISSUE IN ENGLAND AND WALES DURING 1968–78

NUMBER OF DEATHS DURING 1968–78 AND AVERAGE ANNUAL DEATH RATES PER MILLION BY SEX AND AGE GROUPS

AGE GROUP (YEARS)	MEN		WOMEN	
	NUMBER OF DEATHS	RATE PER MILLION	NUMBER OF DEATHS	RATE PER MILLION
0	7	2	3	1
1–4	22	1	32	2
5–14	62	1	45	1
15–24	97	2	68	2
25–34	96	3	78	2
35–44	144	5	108	3
45–54	211	6	199	6
55–64	349	11	323	10
65–74	421	22	421	16
75+	269	33	438	25
ALL AGES	1,678	6	1,715	6

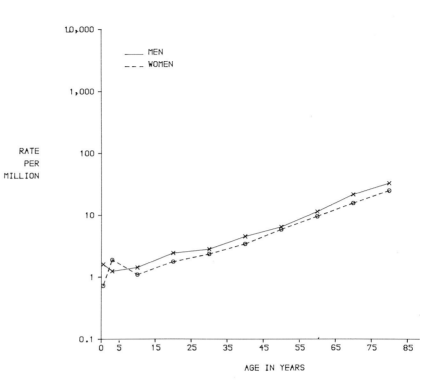

NUMBER OF THE 47 'COUNTY' AREAS SHOWN ON MAP BY LEVEL OF THE STANDARDISED MORTALITY RATIO (SMR) DURING 1968–78

STANDARDISED MORTALITY RATIO	NUMBER OF AREAS	
	MEN	WOMEN
125 AND OVER	6	5
110–124	11	9
90–109	18	17
75–89	7	13
UNDER 75	5	3
LOWEST SMR	37.4	68.6
HIGHEST SMR	200.6	135.0
NUMBER OF AREAS WITH ZERO DEATHS	0	0

MORTALITY FROM MELANOMA OF THE SKIN
IN ENGLAND AND WALES DURING 1968–78

NUMBER OF DEATHS DURING 1968–78 AND AVERAGE ANNUAL
DEATH RATES PER MILLION BY SEX AND AGE GROUPS

AGE GROUP (YEARS)	MEN		WOMEN	
	NUMBER OF DEATHS	RATE PER MILLION	NUMBER OF DEATHS	RATE PER MILLION
0	0	0.0	0	0.0
1–4	1	0.1	1	0.1
5–14	3	0.1	3	0.1
15–24	65	2	93	2
25–34	246	7	246	7
35–44	405	13	468	15
45–54	590	18	782	23
55–64	745	25	851	25
65–74	618	32	787	30
75+	355	44	783	45
ALL AGES	3,028	12	4,014	15

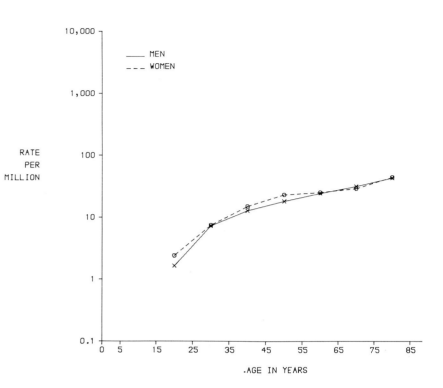

NUMBER OF THE 47 'COUNTY' AREAS SHOWN ON MAP BY LEVEL OF
THE STANDARDISED MORTALITY RATIO (SMR) DURING 1968–78

STANDARDISED MORTALITY RATIO	NUMBER OF AREAS	
	MEN	WOMEN
125 AND OVER	12	7
110–124	7	9
90–109	14	13
75–89	11	16
UNDER 75	3	2
LOWEST SMR	65.3	60.9
HIGHEST SMR	205.7	139.4
NUMBER OF AREAS WITH ZERO DEATHS	0	0

MORTALITY FROM OTHER CANCER OF THE SKIN
IN ENGLAND AND WALES DURING 1968–78

NUMBER OF DEATHS DURIN. ̂8–78 AND AVERAGE ANNUAL
DEATH RATES PER MILLIC. ̂ SEX AND AGE GROUPS

AGE GROUP (YEARS)	MEN		WOMEN	
	NUMBER OF DEATHS	RATE PER MILLION	NUMBER OF DEATHS	RATE PER MILLION
0	1	0.2	0	0.0
1–4	1	0.1	2	0.1
5–14	3	0.1		0.1
15–24	6	0.2	5	0.1
25–34	13	0.4	9	0.3
35–44	41	1	34	1
45–54	194	6	107	
55–64	471	15	284	ε
65–74	818	42	551	21
75+	1,130	139	1,428	82
ALL AGES	2,678	10	2,424	9

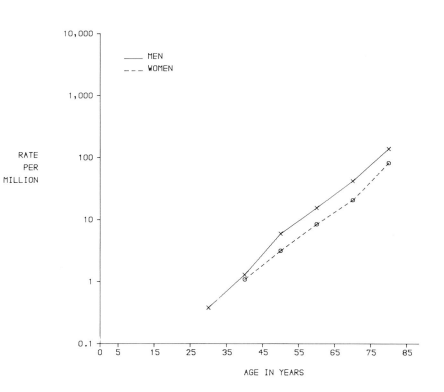

NUMBER OF THE 47 'COUNTY' AREAS SHOWN C ̂ IAP BY LEVEL OF
THE STANDARDISED MORTALITY RATIO (SMR) L ̂ NG 1968–78

STANDARDISED MORTALITY RATIO	NUMBE. ̂ AREAS	
	MEN	WOMEN
125 AND OVER	6	ς
110–124	14	ι
90–109	12	16
75–89	7	7
UNDER 75	8	6
LOWEST SMR	64.4	55.3
HIGHEST SMR	149.0	173.0
NUMBER OF AREAS WITH ZERO DEATHS	0	0

MORTALITY FROM CANCER OF THE VULVA AND OTHER FEMALE GENITAL ORGANS IN ENGLAND AND WALES DURING 1968–78

NUMBER OF DEATHS DURING 1968–78 AND AVERAGE ANNUAL DEATH RATES PER MILLION BY SEX AND AGE GROUPS

AGE GROUP (YEARS)	MEN		WOMEN	
	NUMBER OF DEATHS	RATE PER MILLION	NUMBER OF DEATHS	RATE PER MILLION
0	—	—	1	0.2
1–4	—	—	5	0.3
5–14	—	—	1	0.0
15–24	—	—	4	0.1
25–34	—	—	11	0.3
35–44	—	—	79	3
45–54	—	—	309	9
55–64	—	—	814	24
65–74	—	—	1,751	66
75+	—	—	3,007	173
ALL AGES	—	—	5,982	22

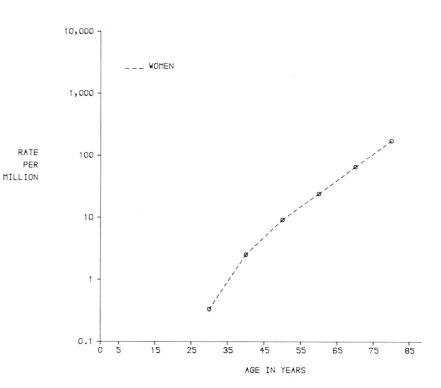

NUMBER OF THE 47 'COUNTY' AREAS SHOWN ON MAP BY LEVEL OF THE STANDARDISED MORTALITY RATIO (SMR) DURING 1968–78

STANDARDISED MORTALITY RATIO	NUMBER OF AREAS	
	MEN	WOMEN
125 AND OVER	—	4
110–124	—	8
90–109	—	23
75–89	—	11
UNDER 75	—	1
LOWEST SMR	—	68.2
HIGHEST SMR	—	146.9
NUMBER OF AREAS WITH ZERO DEATHS	—	0

MORTALITY FROM CANCER OF THE TESTIS
IN ENGLAND AND WALES DURING 1968–78

NUMBER OF DEATHS DURING 1968–78 AND AVERAGE ANNUAL
DEATH RATES PER MILLION BY SEX AND AGE GROUPS

AGE GROUP (YEARS)	MEN		WOMEN	
	NUMBER OF DEATHS	RATE PER MILLION	NUMBER OF DEATHS	RATE PER MILLION
0	0	0.0	—	—
1–4	34	2	—	—
5–14	24	1	—	—
15–24	458	12	—	—
25–34	858	25	—	—
35–44	516	16	—	—
45–54	286	9	—	—
55–64	224	7	—	—
65–74	220	11	—	—
75+	136	17	—	—
ALL AGES	2,756	11	—	—

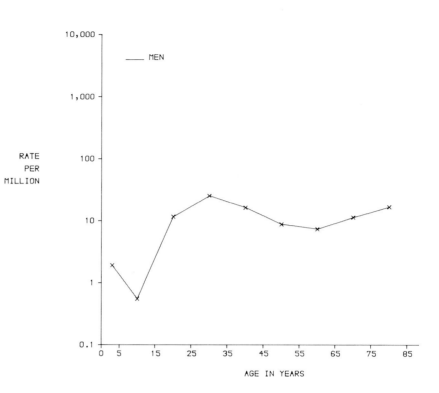

NUMBER OF THE 47 'COUNTY' AREAS SHOWN ON MAP BY LEVEL OF
THE STANDARDISED MORTALITY RATIO (SMR) DURING 1968–78

STANDARDISED MORTALITY RATIO	NUMBER OF AREAS	
	MEN	WOMEN
125 AND OVER	6	—
110–124	8	—
90–109	23	—
75–89	9	—
UNDER 75	1	—
LOWEST SMR	33.9	—
HIGHEST SMR	163.9	—
NUMBER OF AREAS WITH ZERO DEATHS	0	—

MORTALITY FROM CANCER OF THE KIDNEY AND OTHER URINARY ORGANS
IN ENGLAND AND WALES DURING 1968-78

NUMBER OF DEATHS DURING 1968-78 AND AVERAGE ANNUAL
DEATH RATES PER MILLION BY SEX AND AGE GROUPS

AGE GROUP (YEARS)	MEN		WOMEN	
	NUMBER OF DEATHS	RATE PER MILLION	NUMBER OF DEATHS	RATE PER MILLION
0	18	4	9	2
1-4	114	6	109	6
5-14	70	2	100	2
15-24	32	1	28	1
25-34	98	3	59	2
35-44	399	13	186	6
45-54	1,439	44	637	19
55-64	3,172	104	1,509	45
65-74	3,761	195	2,200	83
75+	2,009	248	2,159	124
ALL AGES	11,112	43	6,996	25

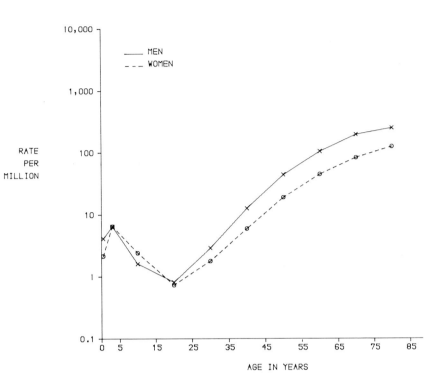

NUMBER OF THE 47 'COUNTY' AREAS SHOWN ON MAP BY LEVEL OF
THE STANDARDISED MORTALITY RATIO (SMR) DURING 1968-78

STANDARDISED MORTALITY RATIO	NUMBER OF AREAS	
	MEN	WOMEN
125 AND OVER	1	3
110-124	2	4
90-109	32	27
75-89	11	11
UNDER 75	1	2
LOWEST SMR	73.5	62.2
HIGHEST SMR	132.6	137.5
NUMBER OF AREAS WITH ZERO DEATHS	0	0

MORTALITY FROM CANCER OF THE BRAIN
IN ENGLAND AND WALES DURING 1968–78

NUMBER OF DEATHS DURING 1968–78 AND AVERAGE ANNUAL DEATH RATES PER MILLION BY SEX AND AGE GROUPS

AGE GROUP (YEARS)	MEN		WOMEN	
	NUMBER OF DEATHS	RATE PER MILLION	NUMBER OF DEATHS	RATE PER MILLION
0	28	6	25	6
1–4	208	12	152	9
5–14	518	12	362	9
15–24	316	8	271	7
25–34	651	19	423	13
35–44	1,234	39	750	24
45–54	2,561	79	1,722	51
55–64	3,854	127	2,703	80
65–74	2,296	119	1,850	69
75+	321	40	381	22
ALL AGES	11,987	46	8,639	31

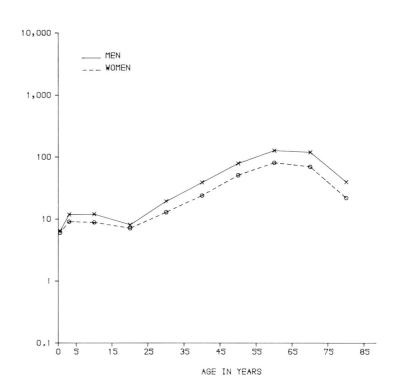

NUMBER OF THE 47 'COUNTY' AREAS SHOWN ON MAP BY LEVEL OF THE STANDARDISED MORTALITY RATIO (SMR) DURING 1968–78

STANDARDISED MORTALITY RATIO	NUMBER OF AREAS	
	MEN	WOMEN
125 AND OVER	2	3
110–124	10	9
90–109	29	23
75–89	4	11
UNDER 75	2	1
LOWEST SMR	53.8	70.2
HIGHEST SMR	134.8	141.9
NUMBER OF AREAS WITH ZERO DEATHS	0	0

MORTALITY FROM CANCER OF THE THYROID GLAND
IN ENGLAND AND WALES DURING 1968–78

NUMBER OF DEATHS DURING 1968–78 AND AVERAGE ANNUAL
DEATH RATES PER MILLION BY SEX AND AGE GROUPS

AGE GROUP (YEARS)	MEN		WOMEN	
	NUMBER OF DEATHS	RATE PER MILLION	NUMBER OF DEATHS	RATE PER MILLION
0	0	0.0	0	0.0
1–4	0	0.0	0	0.0
5–14	0	0.0	1	0.0
15–24	6	0.2	8	0.2
25–34	16	0.5	14	0.4
35–44	45	1	62	2
45–54	147	5	214	6
55–64	311	10	623	19
65–74	436	23	1,007	38
75+	287	35	1,322	76
ALL AGES	1,248	5	3,251	12

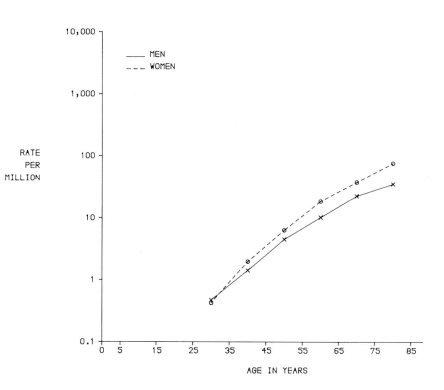

NUMBER OF THE 47 'COUNTY' AREAS SHOWN ON MAP BY LEVEL OF
THE STANDARDISED MORTALITY RATIO (SMR) DURING 1968–78

STANDARDISED MORTALITY RATIO	NUMBER OF AREAS	
	MEN	WOMEN
125 AND OVER	6	1
110–124	7	8
90–109	18	28
75–89	7	7
UNDER 75	9	3
LOWEST SMR	27.0	59.9
HIGHEST SMR	161.7	168.1
NUMBER OF AREAS WITH ZERO DEATHS	0	0

MORTALITY FROM CANCER OF UNSPECIFIED SITE
IN ENGLAND AND WALES DURING 1968–78

NUMBER OF DEATHS DURING 1968–78 AND AVERAGE ANNUAL
DEATH RATES PER MILLION BY SEX AND AGE GROUPS

AGE GROUP (YEARS)	MEN		WOMEN	
	NUMBER OF DEATHS	RATE PER MILLION	NUMBER OF DEATHS	RATE PER MILLION
0	2	0.5	0	0.0
1–4	4	0.2	8	0.5
5–14	13	0.3	11	0.3
15–24	62	2	33	1
25–34	110	3	86	3
35–44	309	10	334	11
45–54	1,215	37	1,225	36
55–64	3,451	114	2,937	87
65–74	5,348	277	4,820	181
75+	3,732	461	6,230	358
ALL AGES	14,246	55	15,684	57

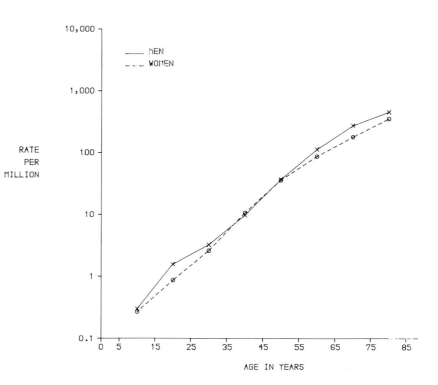

NUMBER OF THE 47 'COUNTY' AREAS SHOWN ON MAP BY LEVEL OF
THE STANDARDISED MORTALITY RATIO (SMR) DURING 1968–78

STANDARDISED MORTALITY RATIO	NUMBER OF AREAS	
	MEN	WOMEN
125 AND OVER	1	2
110–124	6	7
90–109	25	25
75–89	8	8
UNDER 75	7	5
LOWEST SMR	51.3	50.3
HIGHEST SMR	127.5	128.0
NUMBER OF AREAS WITH ZERO DEATHS	0	0

MORTALITY FROM NON-HODGKIN'S LYMPHOMA
IN ENGLAND AND WALES DURING 1968–78

NUMBER OF DEATHS DURING 1968–78 AND AVERAGE ANNUAL DEATH RATES PER MILLION BY SEX AND AGE GROUPS

AGE GROUP (YEARS)	MEN		WOMEN	
	NUMBER OF DEATHS	RATE PER MILLION	NUMBER OF DEATHS	RATE PER MILLION
0	9	2	3	1
1–4	90	5	50	3
5–14	322	7	115	3
15–24	353	9	166	4
25–34	438	13	236	7
35–44	670	21	377	12
45–54	1,383	42	942	28
55–64	2,540	84	1,769	53
65–74	3,010	156	2,759	104
75+	1,715	212	2,590	149
ALL AGES	10,530	40	9,007	33

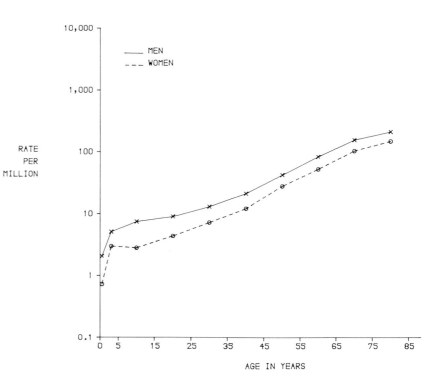

NUMBER OF THE 47 'COUNTY' AREAS SHOWN ON MAP BY LEVEL OF THE STANDARDISED MORTALITY RATIO (SMR) DURING 1968–78

STANDARDISED MORTALITY RATIO	NUMBER OF AREAS	
	MEN	WOMEN
125 AND OVER	0	1
110–124	12	13
90–109	22	19
75–89	10	11
UNDER 75	3	3
LOWEST SMR	58.6	65.6
HIGHEST SMR	124.9	131.4
NUMBER OF AREAS WITH ZERO DEATHS	0	0

MORTALITY FROM HODGKIN'S DISEASE
IN ENGLAND AND WALES DURING 1968–78

NUMBER OF DEATHS DURING 1968–78 AND AVERAGE ANNUAL DEATH RATES PER MILLION BY SEX AND AGE GROUPS

AGE GROUP (YEARS)	MEN		WOMEN	
	NUMBER OF DEATHS	RATE PER MILLION	NUMBER OF DEATHS	RATE PER MILLION
0	0	0.0	0	0.0
1–4	3	0.2	1	0.1
5–14	67	2	23	1
15–24	432	11	274	7
25–34	760	22	388	12
35–44	687	22	335	11
45–54	802	25	391	12
55–64	1,092	36	565	17
65–74	942	49	774	29
75+	390	48	625	36
ALL AGES	5,175	20	3,376	12

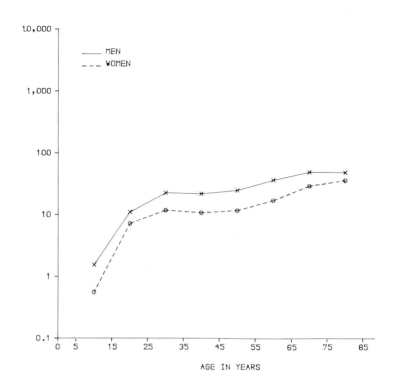

NUMBER OF THE 47 'COUNTY' AREAS SHOWN ON MAP BY LEVEL OF THE STANDARDISED MORTALITY RATIO (SMR) DURING 1968–78

STANDARDISED MORTALITY RATIO	NUMBER OF AREAS	
	MEN	WOMEN
125 AND OVER	5	2
110–124	10	16
90–109	19	15
75–89	11	10
UNDER 75	2	4
LOWEST SMR	62.0	41.5
HIGHEST SMR	134.3	178.0
NUMBER OF AREAS WITH ZERO DEATHS	0	0

MORTALITY FROM MULTIPLE MYELOMA
IN ENGLAND AND WALES DURING 1968–78

NUMBER OF DEATHS DURING 1968–78 AND AVERAGE ANNUAL
DEATH RATES PER MILLION BY SEX AND AGE GROUPS

AGE GROUP (YEARS)	MEN		WOMEN	
	NUMBER OF DEATHS	RATE PER MILLION	NUMBER OF DEATHS	RATE PER MILLION
0	0	0.0	0	0.0
1–4	0	0.0	0	0.0
5–14	0	0.0	0	0.0
15–24	1	0.0	3	0.1
25–34	22	1	10	0.3
35–44	159	5	98	3
45–54	680	21	474	14
55–64	1,839	60	1,435	43
65–74	2,389	124	2,581	97
75+	1,467	181	2,292	132
ALL AGES	6,557	25	6,893	25

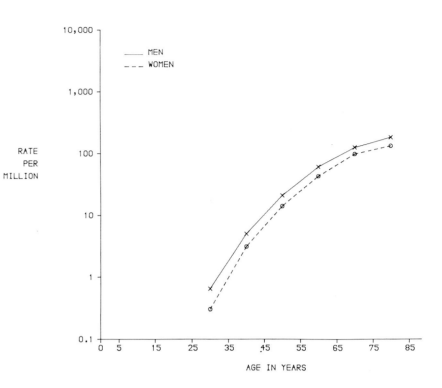

NUMBER OF THE 47 'COUNTY' AREAS SHOWN ON MAP BY LEVEL OF
THE STANDARDISED MORTALITY RATIO (SMR) DURING 1968–78

STANDARDISED MORTALITY RATIO	NUMBER OF AREAS	
	MEN	WOMEN
125 AND OVER	1	3
110–124	8	8
90–109	28	31
75–89	7	5
UNDER 75	3	0
LOWEST SMR	63.5	79.2
HIGHEST SMR	130.0	137.4
NUMBER OF AREAS WITH ZERO DEATHS	0	0

MORTALITY FROM ACUTE LYMPHATIC LEUKAEMIA
IN ENGLAND AND WALES DURING 1968-78

NUMBER OF DEATHS DURING 1968-78 AND AVERAGE ANNUAL DEATH RATES PER MILLION BY SEX AND AGE GROUPS

AGE GROUP (YEARS)	MEN		WOMEN	
	NUMBER OF DEATHS	RATE PER MILLION	NUMBER OF DEATHS	RATE PER MILLION
0	32	7	16	4
1-4	368	21	259	15
5-14	866	20	545	13
15-24	358	9	182	5
25-34	137	4	67	2
35-44	102	3	68	2
45-54	109	3	90	3
55-64	221	7	142	4
65-74	280	15	218	8
75+	237	29	259	15
ALL AGES	2,710	10	1,846	7

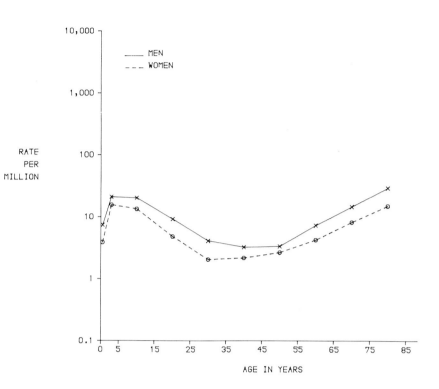

NUMBER OF THE 47 'COUNTY' AREAS SHOWN ON MAP BY LEVEL OF THE STANDARDISED MORTALITY RATIO (SMR) DURING 1968-78

STANDARDISED MORTALITY RATIO	NUMBER OF AREAS	
	MEN	WOMEN
125 AND OVER	9	10
110-124	5	7
90-109	19	14
75-89	9	12
UNDER 75	5	4
LOWEST SMR	50.7	36.4
HIGHEST SMR	151.8	175.3
NUMBER OF AREAS WITH ZERO DEATHS	0	0

MORTALITY FROM CHRONIC LYMPHATIC LEUKAEMIA
IN ENGLAND AND WALES DURING 1968–78

NUMBER OF DEATHS DURING 1968–78 AND AVERAGE ANNUAL DEATH RATES PER MILLION BY SEX AND AGE GROUPS

AGE GROUP (YEARS)	MEN		WOMEN	
	NUMBER OF DEATHS	RATE PER MILLION	NUMBER OF DEATHS	RATE PER MILLION
0	0	0.0	0	0.0
1–4	2	0.1	2	0.1
5–14	15	0.3	6	0.1
15–24	5	0.1	4	0.1
25–34	9	0.3	7	0.2
35–44	31	1	12	0.4
45–54	240	7	99	3
55–64	866	28	386	11
65–74	1,622	84	871	33
75+	1,483	183	1,712	98
ALL AGES	4,273	16	3,099	11

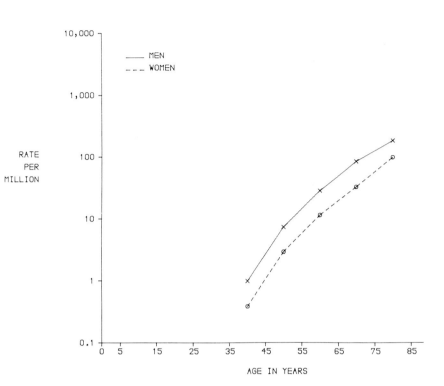

NUMBER OF THE 47 'COUNTY' AREAS SHOWN ON MAP BY LEVEL OF THE STANDARDISED MORTALITY RATIO (SMR) DURING 1968–78

STANDARDISED MORTALITY RATIO	NUMBER OF AREAS	
	MEN	WOMEN
125 AND OVER	2	8
110–124	11	4
90–109	21	25
75–89	12	8
UNDER 75	1	2
LOWEST SMR	52.6	55.8
HIGHEST SMR	159.7	180.7
NUMBER OF AREAS WITH ZERO DEATHS	0	0

MORTALITY FROM ACUTE MYELOID LEUKAEMIA
IN ENGLAND AND WALES DURING 1968–78

NUMBER OF DEATHS DURING 1968–78 AND AVERAGE ANNUAL
DEATH RATES PER MILLION BY SEX AND AGE GROUPS

AGE GROUP (YEARS)	MEN		WOMEN	
	NUMBER OF DEATHS	RATE PER MILLION	NUMBER OF DEATHS	RATE PER MILLION
0	20	5	23	6
1–4	98	6	92	5
5–14	216	5	208	5
15–24	362	9	274	7
25–34	333	10	315	10
35–44	440	14	358	11
45–54	671	21	612	18
55–64	1,159	38	890	27
65–74	1,482	77	1,361	51
75+	1,008	124	1,331	77
ALL AGES	5,789	22	5,464	20

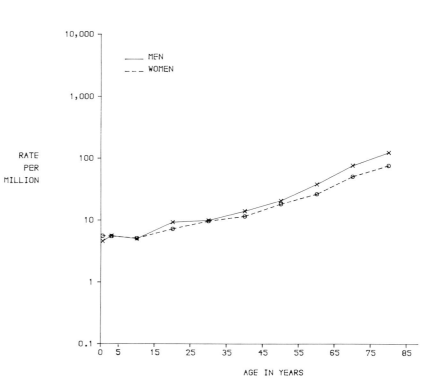

NUMBER OF THE 47 'COUNTY' AREAS SHOWN ON MAP BY LEVEL OF
THE STANDARDISED MORTALITY RATIO (SMR) DURING 1968–78

STANDARDISED MORTALITY RATIO	NUMBER OF AREAS	
	MEN	WOMEN
125 AND OVER	1	2
110–124	8	7
90–109	25	23
75–89	10	12
UNDER 75	3	3
LOWEST SMR	51.3	46.1
HIGHEST SMR	126.1	137.3
NUMBER OF AREAS WITH ZERO DEATHS	0	0

MORTALITY FROM CHRONIC MYELOID LEUKAEMIA
IN ENGLAND AND WALES DURING 1968–78

NUMBER OF DEATHS DURING 1968–78 AND AVERAGE ANNUAL
DEATH RATES PER MILLION BY SEX AND AGE GROUPS

AGE GROUP (YEARS)	MEN		WOMEN	
	NUMBER OF DEATHS	RATE PER MILLION	NUMBER OF DEATHS	RATE PER MILLION
0	3	1	0	0.0
1–4	19	1	10	1
5–14	27	1	17	0.4
15–24	62	2	45	1
25–34	146	4	108	3
35–44	214	7	177	6
45–54	382	12	335	10
55–64	572	19	544	16
65–74	823	43	734	28
75+	685	85	869	50
ALL AGES	2,933	11	2,839	10

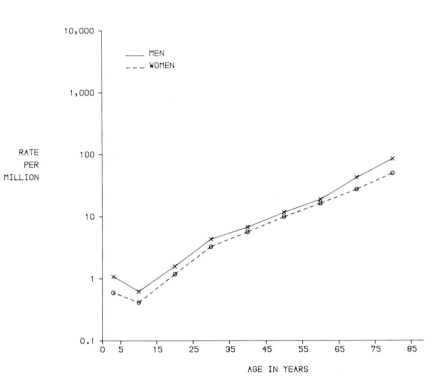

NUMBER OF THE 47 'COUNTY' AREAS SHOWN ON MAP BY LEVEL OF
THE STANDARDISED MORTALITY RATIO (SMR) DURING 1968–78

STANDARDISED MORTALITY RATIO	NUMBER OF AREAS	
	MEN	WOMEN
125 AND OVER	4	5
110–124	10	8
90–109	20	19
75–89	7	6
UNDER 75	6	9
LOWEST SMR	41.5	57.8
HIGHEST SMR	133.4	148.9
NUMBER OF AREAS WITH ZERO DEATHS	0	0